PRAISE FOR
THE BODYMIND BALLWORK METHOD

"*The Bodymind Ballwork Method* is very compatible with yoga practices, as well as with other forms of bodywork therapy. What I like most about the book is how elegantly Saltonstall explains the science behind the movements she teaches, while revealing how our unfolding consciousness on the balls is an integral part of this healing modality."

—JUDITH HANSON LASATER, PhD, PT, yoga teacher, and author of nine books, including *Restore and Rebalance: Yoga for Deep Relaxation*

"Ellen Saltonstall is a teacher of integrity who puts her arms confidently around her subject and delivers a clear path for improving interoceptive awareness. A terrific adjunct to any movement practice."

—TOM MYERS, author of *Anatomy Trains*

"After a lifetime exploring embodiment, I appreciate Saltonstall's enthusiastic embrace of embodied self-awareness as a key to healing. The effective and easy-to-understand chapters on awareness, stress, trauma, the nervous system, and peripheral receptors place each of the beautifully detailed and illustrated ballwork exercises in a clear conceptual and embodied context."

—ALAN FOGEL, professor of psychology emeritus at the University of Utah, Rosen Method Bodywork practitioner and senior teacher, and author of *Body Sense: The Science and Practice of Embodied Self-Awareness*

"Ellen Saltonstall has written a comprehensive, yet concise, guide to the wonderful world of ballwork. She covers much more than technique (though she does that too!) giving the reader a way into a deeper level of awareness and embodied knowledge."

—CARRIE OWERKO, senior certified teacher of Iyengar Yoga and Laban Movement analyst

"Nobody needs to live in chronic pain. Ellen Saltonstall is a veteran in her field and has been using ballwork long before it became popular. Her vast knowledge of anatomy and movement is compiled in this book. The reader can either dive deep into the foundations of bodymind connection and/or choose to explore the ball exercises for his or her individual needs. The rewards are great, and a feeling of empowerment and lightness arises when chronic pain disappears after doing one of her routines. Self-myofascial release allows a person to take their life back into their own hands. Whether you are a beginner or an athlete or a person in constant chronic pain this book is for you."

—SIMONE LINDNER, Structural Integration practitioner

THE BODYMIND BALLWORK METHOD

A Self-Directed Practice to Help You
Move with Ease, Release Tension, and
Relieve Chronic Pain

Ellen Saltonstall

North Atlantic Books
Berkeley, California

Published by
North Atlantic Books
Berkeley, California

Cover photos by Paula Court and Ellen Saltonstall
Cover design by Emma Cofod
Interior design by Happenstance Type-O-Rama
Illustrations by Emily Ciosek

The Bodymind Ballwork Method: A Self-Directed Practice to Help You Move with Ease, Release Tension, and Relieve Chronic Pain is sponsored and published by the Society for the Study of Native Arts and Sciences (dba North Atlantic Books), an educational nonprofit based in Berkeley, California, that collaborates with partners to develop cross-cultural perspectives, nurture holistic views of art, science, the humanities, and healing, and seed personal and global transformation by publishing work on the relationship of body, spirit, and nature.

North Atlantic Books' publications are available through most bookstores. For further information, visit our website at www.northatlanticbooks.com or call 800-733-3000.

Library of Congress Cataloguing-in-Publication data is available from the publisher upon request.

1 2 3 4 5 6 7 8 9 Sheridan 22 21 20 19 18

Printed on recycled paper

North Atlantic Books is committed to the protection of our environment. We partner with FSC-certified printers using soy-based inks and print on recycled paper whenever possible.

CONTENTS

PHOTO CREDITS

All illustrations other than photographs by Emily Ciosek

ACKNOWLEDGMENTS

Thanks to my parents for their unconditional support of me and for the values of diligence, honesty, and generosity by which they lived. From decades of my professional life in dance, yoga, and bodywork, I have been inspired by many teachers, notably Elaine Summers, Merce Cunningham, Anahid Sofian, Twyla Tharp, John Friend, Thomas Myers, Judith Lasater, Mary Dunn, and Carrie Owerko—their fascination with movement is contagious. My students and clients have supported me, challenged me, and fueled me to continue learning. The Bodymind Ballwork method is greatly enriched and inspired by their questions and explorations over many years and in many contexts. I'm particularly grateful for the students who gave permission for their stories to be told in this book.

I heartily applaud the growing community of bodywork professionals, neurologists, and psychotherapists who are forging an ever-new understanding of the bodymind connection. They are pioneers, integrating the scientific, psychological, and spiritual perspectives of who we are as humans, and highlighting the incredible healing potential of this kind of practice. Many of them are represented by quotes within this text, and by their books that are listed in the bibliography at the end of this book.

Thanks to those who modeled for the photographs in this book: Susan Genis, Lucia McBee, Yukiko Matsubara, Joyce Cohen, Eduardo Martinez, and Nick Fitch. Thanks to the photographers Paula Court, John Pilson, and Josef Kushner, and to the illustrator Emily Ciosek. David Fink generously provided comments and suggestions as I developed this book. Thanks to editors Julia Hough and Miriam Seidel, whose word skills helped me to shape this book.

As this project came to fruition, my literary agent Jill Marsal found a home for it at North Atlantic Books, where editor Pam Berkman has been its skillful shepherd through the editorial process. I appreciate their expertise in helping me to refine what I have to say.

Lastly, special thanks goes to my family for their constant love and support.

INTRODUCTION

There is a unity of experience—of one experience with another and all experiences together—in which all the thousand-fold occurrences in life become inseparably connected. This unity must be so fully thought through that it becomes an essential part of the person, by which she/he is led intuitively in every moment.[1]

We each live in our own version of this magnificently complex and capable human body. We eat, sleep, play, and work, seeking discovery and satisfaction in one way or another. The body is our constant companion and a large part of who we are. But do we really feel it, appreciate it, and have an ongoing dialogue with it? This book explores the bodymind relationship and describes how we can practice a method of self-care that is simple yet profound.

Does your body feel like a burden, an enemy, a dangerous mystery, or an ally and a reservoir of knowledge? When you have pain or restrictions in your body, do you turn to others for help because your body is "acting up"? Can you listen to what wisdom might be right there under your skin? The body's intelligence is separate from our IQ, our education, and our intellect, all of which have taken on a higher value in modern culture. We need to give our body intelligence more opportunities to shine.

In my career as a massage therapist and teacher of body awareness and yoga, I have come to appreciate and value the process of staying in touch with the ever-present connection between my body and my mind, and helping my students to do the same. This means being aware of physical sensations and emotions with an attitude of nonjudgmental curiosity and attentiveness. I see how my experience in my body at any given moment is a fundamental support and resource for self-knowledge in a larger sense. The body has its own language, which we are born knowing but which for many reasons is often forgotten. Teaching students to relearn this language has been immensely rewarding to me. This type of study and practice is often referred to as "somatics"; the word *soma* (from the Greek and Sanskrit) means the "body perceived from within."

Throughout history, self-awareness and holistic healing methods have offered seekers the tools to know themselves better and live healthier lives. Yoga and other age-old Eastern movement arts like Aikido, Qi Gong, and Tai Chi teach that the life force energy (fueling both body and mind) can be regulated and enhanced by disciplined practice. During the twentieth century many wonderful techniques emerged that help people to become more aware of who they are. Some are therapies in which a practitioner works on you and you are relatively passive, as in the many types of manual therapy. Others place emphasis on physical alignment and healthy movement patterns, such as the Alexander Technique, Feldenkrais Method, Ideokinesis, Body-Mind Centering, and Sensory Awareness. Still others draw direct attention to the bodymind connection in a more psychological direction. These include Phoenix Rising Yoga Therapy, Rosen Method Bodywork and Movement, and Somatics.[2] Through parallel and often overlapping pathways, these pioneering methods have given us tools to learn more authentically who we are—what "human nature" really is.

Bodymind Ballwork is a method that starts with the body, by feeling and massaging the muscles and fascia with pressure from rubber balls. It seems simple, doesn't it? Self-massage using these tools that are really toys. But wonderful things happen. Chronic and acute physical pain can be relieved—often quite quickly. I frequently hear the lower back, hips, neck, and shoulders mentioned as trouble spots that have been relieved. More ease of movement and breathing are other perks that students experience right from the very beginning.

But what also develops gradually as practice continues over time is an opening in the inner dialogue between body and mind, and a profound investigation of self-awareness. We start to understand how there can really be no separation between body and mind—that every sensory experience has an emotional correlate, and every emotion and thought pattern is imprinted into our physical tissues in some way. The body reveals patterns of sensation, which then reveal patterns of thought and emotion. The body begins to teach its language to us, starting wherever we are. Some come to this work already attuned to inner sensations, but for others, it's entirely new territory.

We all have at least some self-awareness—we know when we are tired, hungry, happy, or sad. We recognize pain and possibly fear when we get injured. Hopefully we enjoy sensual pleasure. Self-awareness has two complementary forms: conceptual self-awareness and embodied self-awareness.[3] Conceptual self-awareness is made up of our cognitive thoughts about ourselves, with associated memories, observations, evaluations, and analysis. It includes autobiographical memory, pleasure seeking, and goal setting. Thoughts such as "My body has a certain size and shape," "My personality has these traits," or "My history includes these stories" show us thinking of ourselves as "object." Talking psychotherapy relies on this type of self-awareness in the journey, and there is tremendous benefit in exploring our self-knowledge verbally in this way.

Embodied self-awareness is the "feeling" state without analysis—in other words, being the "subject." Ask yourself: What is my sensory and emotional experience right now? What is happening in my body, my breath, and my mind? Can I feel my body position, my breath, my state of attention, my energy level? This kind of awareness is not dependent on language. It exists only in the present moment, and it doesn't need any rationale, explanation, or strategy. It is simply what and who we are right now. Typically we are not educated to develop this type of awareness; we are socialized from a very young age to behave in certain ways without noticing what we "feel." Yet embodied self-awareness is crucial to taking good care of ourselves, even if it does not follow societal norms. As Alan Fogel states so succinctly in the preface to his book *Body Sense,* "Awareness is medicine."[4]

Embodied self-awareness helps us to notice possible physical and emotional issues before they escalate. Athletes and dancers can prevent and treat injuries; older students can improve coordination and balance to avoid falls; and hardworking folks of all ages and all professions can relieve the aches and pains—and mental stress—of a demanding life. People who already receive massage, chiropractic care, or physical therapy can augment and support their treatments by using the balls at home between sessions. Bodymind Ballwork has the potential to lessen the symptoms of common chronic ailments such as stress-related cardiovascular disease, immune dysfunction, and depression in ways that can be life-changing.

However, embodied self-awareness is easy to lose, with our modern culture's priorities on medical interventions for body problems, and reliance on technology and outside "experts" to deal with health issues. We forget that we each live in our own body, and therefore we have the best chance of under-standing it. Embodied self-awareness doesn't come without some effort; it must be actively practiced, cultivated, and maintained as a self-directed path of dis-covery in order to serve its purpose of helping us attain our best state of health.

Psychologist Bessel van der Kolk, in his book *The Body Keeps the Score*, says it this way:

> If you are not aware of what your body needs, you can't take care of it. If you don't feel hunger, you can't nourish yourself. If you mistake anxiety for hunger, you may eat too much. And if you can't feel when you're satiated, you'll keep eating. Most traditional therapies down-play or ignore the moment-to-moment shifts in our inner sensory world. But these shifts carry the essence of the organism's response: the emotional states that are imprinted in the body's chemical profile, in the viscera, in the contraction of the striated muscles of the face, throat, trunk and limbs…. Once you start approaching your body with curiosity rather than with fear, everything shifts.[5]

Joan, a psychotherapist, learned about the ballwork while studying yoga with me. It appealed to her as a noninvasive and effective way to deal with the various physical problems she was having at the time—sacroiliac dysfunction, lower back spasms, and plantar fasciitis. She wrote of her first experience: "It was love at first sight! It felt like getting an expert Shiatsu massage, but one in which I could control the location, intensity, and duration of the massage myself." As she began to work on the areas of greatest need, other insights emerged. She realized that a fall three years before had caused her chest and ribs to tighten, which significantly affected her lower back and pelvis. As she began to work with the balls on her chest, her breathing became fuller and deeper. She says: "I find the ballwork to be both exciting and soothing—mentally, physically, and spiritually. It helps me fix most of the problems I used to go to doctors for. Spending time taking good care of myself feels like a gift, and gives me control of my life as I age. Having tools to keep myself active and mobile is so reassuring. It's also helpful for mood regulation. Whether I'm feeling speedy or lethargic, using a ball on my spine for ten minutes totally recenters me."

Linda owns and operates a horse riding and training facility. She says:

> I have fallen off horses and done heavy, repetitive manual chores for twenty years, which has resulted in chronic pain not relieved by massage, chiropractic, or electrical stimulation. When I met Ellen, I was skeptical of the ballwork at first because it was painful. But Ellen

helped me to modify the degree of pressure so that I could tolerate it, and day by day my muscles and fascia began to loosen. The twenty-year pain behind my shoulder is gone. My plantar fasciitis is gone. The pain in my right buttock is gone. I haven't felt this good since I started working with horses. Since learning this technique I have practiced it every day and I feel wonderful.

Throughout this book, you will meet others like Joan and Linda who practice Bodymind Ballwork. Their stories and reflections offer previews of the treasures this work offers for your well-being throughout your life.

THE LINEAGE OF BODYMIND BALLWORK

As mentioned earlier, the early and mid-twentieth century was a rich time for the development of somatic education. This era saw intensely contrasting trends in education, politics, and culture, with people learning about the ideas of Sigmund Freud, Wilhelm Reich, Karl Marx, and Maria Montessori, all at the same time Hitler was coming into power. In Europe at that time, the prevailing system of physical education was pre-military training for boys and men, emphasizing muscle building, calisthenics, and competitive sports. In response to that, several women in Germany introduced a different approach for girls and women called Gymnastik, with the purpose of fostering development of natural movement, coordination, rhythm, and emotional expression. The two main proponents of Gymnastik were Hede Kallmeyer and Bess Mensendieck, both of whom had studied with Genevieve Stebbins (1857-1934), a teacher of the Delsarte method in America.

Although Gymnastik was separate from the public school system in Germany, it became an established (though still revolutionary) professional teaching field, regulated by the government and requiring three years of training. Elsa Gindler (1885-1961) was trained in Gymnastik and became a central figure in her field. Gindler is the unsung pioneer of bodymind work, and her influence has been tremendous. She was interested in the challenge of keeping the body healthy and strong without sacrificing sensitivity and curiosity, and nurturing a sense of exploration of the capacities of our human body and mind. She called her work "Arbeit am Menschen," or "work on the human being."

As often happens with innovators, Gindler developed her original work in response to her own needs. In her twenties she had been diagnosed with incurable tuberculosis. Instead of the retreat to breathe pure mountain air that her doctors recommended, she decided to do her own deep inner work to develop her own body's healing powers. She worked patiently and persistently with her breathing, and in a year she was cured. What she learned became the basis of her life's work. Gindler documented her work extensively, but all her records were destroyed when a bomb hit her studio just before the end of World War II–a devastating loss.

Here are a few excerpts from "Gymnastik for Busy People," her only surviving article, in which Gindler speaks of bodymind unity:

> The aim of my work is not learning certain movements, but rather the achievement of concentration. Only by means of concentration can we attain the full functioning of the physical apparatus in relation to mental and spiritual life. [This work] can only be entered into and understood through consciousness.... By that I mean consciousness that is centered, reacts to the environment, and can think and feel.
>
> Relaxation is that condition in which we have the greatest capacity of reacting. It is a stillness within us, a readiness to respond appropriately to any stimulus.
>
> Whoever is truly able to relax is also capable of healthy tension. This we perceive as the beautiful changeability of energies that react to every stimulus, increasing and diminishing as required. Above all, it includes a strong feeling of inner strength, of effortlessness in accomplishment—in short, a heightened joie de vivre.[6]

Gindler trained many teachers, among them Charlotte Selver and Carola Speads, who both brought her work to America. Others in this "second generation" of somatic educators (not trained by Gindler but aware of or influenced by her work) were F. M. Alexander, Moshe Feldenkrais, Mabel Elsworth Todd, Ida Rolf, Irmgard Bartenieff, and Marion Rosen. Thanks to these pioneers, there are many excellent methods for accessing the healing power of bodymind awareness that are known throughout the world.

As somatic work spread in the worlds of dance, theater, and alternative healing, there was significant cross-fertilization, which continues through today. Elaine Summers (1925-2014) studied with Selver and Speads early in her career as a dancer, choreographer, and filmmaker. Elaine developed the method called Kinetic Awareness, a method of self-awareness using slow movement and ballwork to deepen the practitioner's detailed awareness and articulation of movement. Many dancers and choreographers worked with Elaine as part of their training and self-care, finding the work to be essential for preventing or healing the injuries that are inevitable for dancers. I met Elaine as an injured dancer wanting to get rid of knee pain, and this deep work soon became an integral part of my life as a dancer, massage therapist, and yoga teacher. I am grateful to have worked closely with Elaine over many years, and her teachings continue to resonate in my current work with Bodymind Ballwork.

HOW TO USE THIS BOOK

In part I, we will look at the bodymind connection in some detail. Chapter 1 provides a useful map from the yoga tradition describing the layers of our awareness, making the point that any experience is multilayered and never just in the body or the mind. Chapter 2 looks at the nervous system; if you are curious about how your body accomplishes the tasks of awareness, self-regulation, stress management, and relaxation, this chapter will offer some of the neuroscience of those topics. Chapter 3 includes information about our soft tissues, especially fascia, and how bodywork helps us release tension. In chapter 4 we discuss how we form an "idea" or sense of our body, our posture, and how the power of conditioning influences our perceptions. Chapter 5 looks at some common defense mechanisms and why it is helpful or even essential to address long-held psychological issues with embodied self-awareness.

In part II, chapters 6 through 14 will teach you how to practice Bodymind Ballwork. Chapter 6 outlines some basic principles of the work that are helpful to understand before you start. Chapter 7 gives instructions for the most popular techniques—those that I consider to be "everyday" practices. From there, chapters 8 through 14 outline all the possible ways you can use balls on every part of the body, from head to toes. You can skip directly to these practice chapters in part II if you wish. It is my hope that this book gives you a starting place for a practice that will develop over time. You'll learn by doing it, and the conversation between your bodymind and the balls will guide and teach you.

Chapter 15, the conclusion, reviews the benefits of the work and offers possible applications in education, health care settings, and spiritual disciplines.

It is my hope that bodymind techniques like this one can be integrated into our collective consciousness and health care repertoire. Our own awareness is an untapped resource that is ready to help us live life to the fullest extent possible.

PART I

CHAPTER 1

The Bodymind Connection

It is now a well-accepted understanding that the body and the mind cannot be considered as functionally separate. Daily life demonstrates how they overlap in a multitude of ways. Can you think of instances of having headaches or neck pain when you're under pressure at work, or times when back pain or indigestion makes you irritable or unfocused? The mind and body are in constant dialogue. The past twenty-five years have brought ample research and new understanding of how our physiology affects our emotions, and how stress can contribute to chronic illnesses such as irritable bowel syndrome and heart disease.[1] This chapter will address the bodymind connection from various angles and will illustrate ways in which Bodymind Ballwork can contribute to more than just releasing muscle tension. We will look at questions such as these:

What are some of the mechanisms at work when we lie on the rubber balls to release tension?

How does the practice retrain our nervous system toward greater ease?

How are sensory experiences related to states of mind?

Where and how does our sense of "self" register in the brain?

How can we learn to trust our sensations and our power to heal if we've suffered trauma, fear, or extreme pain in the body?

THE LAYERS OF BEING

Deep awareness work encourages us to feel many layers of our being. From a physiological viewpoint, this means feeling the skin, the connective tissue just under the skin, the layers of muscles, the depth of the joints, the organs, and the connections between everything. We have fascia—surrounding every muscle, every bone, and every organ—that is richly supplied with sensory nerves that are always reporting in. Can we hear those messages? Thanks to the slow, calming pace of the ballwork, we have that opportunity.

Learning to feel those components of the physical body—skin, joints, organs, fascia—is a good beginning to a bodywork practice. But there's so much more to feel and notice. The yoga tradition, which goes back thousands of years, is founded upon the idea of the union of body, mind, and spirit—it is the earliest bodymind discipline we know of. Yoga identifies five layers of our being called **koshas,** or sheaths.[2] The koshas provide a map of what the inner journey can reveal. Just as you'd want a map when visiting a new city or hiking in the mountains, a map can clarify experiences and provide a feeling of security along the way. The system of koshas gives a template of the levels of experience you might have when practicing Bodymind Ballwork or any practice that evokes deep awareness. They are not separate; all five are present everywhere in the body, but for the purpose of understanding we can separate them.

The outermost layer is called **annamaya kosha,** literally the "body of food." This sheath exemplifies that we are what we eat; the food we eat transforms into the cells and tissues of the body. It's also called the "gross" body, since it is tangible. It's the part of our consciousness that includes the five senses—hearing, seeing, touching, tasting, and smelling. This kosha includes **interoception,** the sensations that come from the inside of the body, such as rumbling in your stomach or soreness in your muscles. Clearly, working with the balls and movement calls our attention to this level of being. People often report that they can feel more sensation than they thought was there, as if they are feeling their shoulder or their foot or their neck in a whole new way. The sensory nerves and mechanoreceptors that we have everywhere in the body awaken and tell their stories when given the chance.

The second kosha is **pranamaya kosha,** or the "body of breath." The breath continues without our needing to direct or control it, yet it can be a rich field of exploration while practicing. What sensations accompany your normal breath? Are there parts of your body that seem to restrict your breath? Does your breath feel satisfying and nourishing? People often comment that the ballwork helps to expand the breath, giving the feeling that the body is more available to the breath's natural flow in a very satisfying way. We begin to feel how the breath literally animates the body.

Closely interwoven with the breath is the third kosha, called **manomaya kosha,** the "mental body." This is the kosha of thoughts and emotions. It is housed in the nervous system but resonates in every part of the body. As you practice Bodymind Ballwork, you may get in touch with a stream of consciousness that can feel like a dream, or like watching an internal movie. You may be able to "watch" your mind constantly moving, reflecting on experiences of the past or planning the next part of your day. These reflections and dreams are connected to memories stored in our tissues, so when we work with the balls, those mental images emerge. The slow and quiet nature of the work helps set the conditions for this kind of self-observation of the mind.

The next kosha is **vijnanamaya kosha,** the "wisdom body." When your awareness is in the wisdom body, you *know* beyond the shadow of a doubt. Your mind might still be debating—should I pursue this course of action or that one? But somewhere inside you, you know the answer. Resolutions to large and small dilemmas spontaneously arise, and uncertainties dissolve. This kind of clarity (often at the least predictable times) comes from our wisdom body. Often, when students find an area that has been holding tension and they are able to release it, there is a deep "breath of insight" or "breath of confirmation"[3] when they know that something profound about themselves has been released or revealed. It's liberating and inspiring to discover that we can contact that deep place of knowing.

The last kosha is **anandamaya kosha,** or the "body of bliss," in which we have a spontaneous feeling of deep well-being that is not dependent on outer circumstances. Although it's hard to put into words, it has been described as wholeness, integration, freedom, transcendence, or ecstasy. The yoga tradition teaches that this is our true nature, yet we don't experience it as often as we might like. You have probably had many small experiences of this before, when doing something you love or being with someone you love. In this state, the deepest essence of life pervades our perceptions as we rise above, or penetrate beneath, the fluctuating waves of outer experience. Deep awareness work is one pathway to this body of bliss.

Whether from the yogic viewpoint described above, or from a Western scientific viewpoint, the mind and body are always connected. In the next chapter we'll look at the Western scientific view of how our experiences are processed through the nervous system.

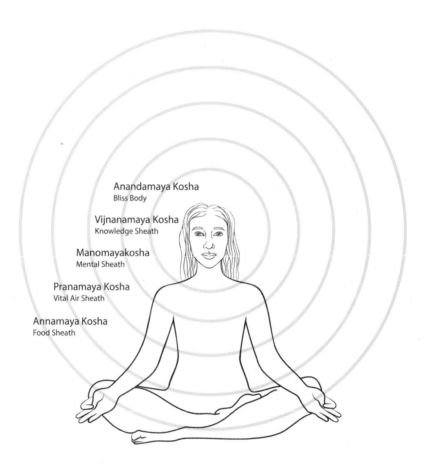

Anandamaya Kosha
Bliss Body

Vijnanamaya Kosha
Knowledge Sheath

Manomayakosha
Mental Sheath

Pranamaya Kosha
Vital Air Sheath

Annamaya Kosha
Food Sheath

The Five Koshas

CHAPTER 2

The Nervous System, Stress, and Relaxation

The biological entry point for our exploration of the koshas is the nervous system, our consciousness. The nervous system is the connecting and integrating link between body and mind, a vast network of communication circuits that coordinates the brain with all the other body systems, sending instantaneous electrical messages throughout the body. We receive information from the world around us, process it, and then choose to take action, all through the nervous system. It governs our heartbeats and breathing, our movements, and our body chemistry, but also our thoughts, intentions, and emotions. Unlike most of the animal kingdom, whose reactions to the environment are instinctual and repetitive, humans can make infinite choices, create art, and learn innumerable skills and ideas—all thanks to the sophistication of our nervous system. We can even learn to modify the functioning of our own nervous system, and this is the great promise of bodywork, meditation, and other bodymind modalities. I'll give a few examples of some parts of the nervous system that characterize a typical day (a complete guide is beyond the scope of this book). This diagram showing the overall map of the nervous system is useful as a reference.

A DAY IN YOUR LIFE

You wake up and remember where and who you are, making the transition from sleep and dreams to alertness. That's the **reticular formation** in your **brainstem,** telling you that you're awake. It is the gateway for stimuli coming from the environment, helping you to respond with appropriate states of alertness or relaxation. We can sleep through city noise, yet awaken to a baby's cry, because of the reticular formation. At night, when we lie still with our eyes closed, especially in a darkened room, the reticular formation signals the body to settle into repose. Other functions of your brainstem (which includes the pons, medulla oblongata, and midbrain) are regulation of your breathing and heart rate, and signals of hunger and thirst. In other words, it's all about basic survival.

So now you're awake and moving. You begin to feel and move your body. Now your **peripheral nerves** (connecting your brain to every part of the body) begin to report in, feeling the touch of the bedclothes, feeling the movement of your limbs as you start to get up. The peripheral nerves are of two types: sensory and motor nerves. The sensory nerves report sensations to the brain (traffic sounds, the smell of coffee, the brightness of light, the temperature of the room, the feeling of the floor under your feet), and the motor nerves stimulate the muscles to contract. Most of the time we're not conscious of many of these messages, but it's possible to become more attuned to them with practice.

Your **cerebral cortex,** the most evolved part of the brain, kicks in when you decide to get up. It organizes your intention, your sensations, your body awareness, and your knowledge of how to interact with your world. There are two hemispheres, or halves, of the cerebral cortex that coordinate with each other through a thick connecting band of nerve fibers called the **corpus callosum.** Despite the popular notion that the two hemispheres have different domains (the left for language and logic, the right for spatial awareness and creativity), we now know that it's not that clear-cut; these functions take place in various regions of the brain. As you get up and walk through your house or apartment, both hemispheres are working together.

Once you are upright, your balance and coordination are governed by your **cerebellum,** which is just above the brainstem. You can consciously attend to balance by using sensors in your feet and all your joints, but a significant part of balancing takes place automatically in the brain.

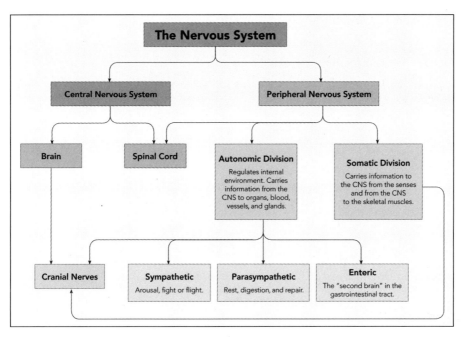

The Nervous System

Perhaps now that you're up, you'll notice your overall energy level. Do you feel calm and quiet, making a slow transition to being awake, or do you feel stimulated to briskly start your day? This sense of the energy level in your mind and body is the function of the **autonomic nervous system (ANS),** which regulates your body and mind from moment to moment below the surface of your everyday awareness. The ANS's functions include your heart rate, your blood pressure, and your metabolism.

The ANS has two divisions, the **sympathetic nervous system (SNS)** and the **parasympathetic nervous system (PNS),** which are always in a balancing act with each other. When we're resting, we are predominantly in the parasympathetic mode, often called the "rest, digest, repair" mode. When we are excited and active, we are in the sympathetic mode, also known as the "fight, flight, or freeze" mode.[1] We fluctuate constantly between these two opposite ends of the energy spectrum, and those fluctuations can be as small as gently waking from sleep, or as large as responding to the sound of gunshots nearby.

I invite you to reflect on whether you tend to spend most of your day in sympathetic mode (stimuli, activity, maybe even anxiety) or in parasympathetic mode (quietness, rest, fatigue, lethargy, or depression). Or perhaps you are balanced: sometimes active, sometimes at rest. The yoga tradition gives a name to that third, balanced state—it's called sattva guna, or harmony and clarity. The three gunas are said to be the three qualities of nature, and we can see any aspect of life through this lens—our work, our self-care, our relationships, our inner dialogue.[2] The **guna of rajas** is the state of activity and excitement at one end of the spectrum, and the **guna of tamas** is the state of rest or inertia at the other end of the spectrum. One goal of yoga practice is to find access to the third state between the two extremes—**sattva guna,** or balance and harmony, on a regular basis. Not that you never get excited, or never sleep—of course life does and should have this whole range of qualities. But often we get stuck in one extreme or the other. Like yoga, Bodymind Ballwork can help to revive you if you are lethargic, and also calm you down if you are agitated, bringing you to the balanced state of sattva guna.

THE STRESS RESPONSE

Because you may be reading this book to learn how to reduce your stress, let's look at the stress response in more detail. Stress is a fact of life, and in moderation it's beneficial for our health. Stress can stimulate us to grow. But if it's experienced in excess and is sustained over the long haul, it's a whole other story.

Stress can be defined as anything that knocks our system out of basic homeostasis. Stress can come from overwork, from past or present trauma, from fear, from illness, from sleep deprivation—the list goes on. Hans Selye (1907-1982), a Hungarian endocrinologist, expanded our understanding of stress. He identified two different types of stress: negative stress, which he called **distress,** and positive stress, which he called **eustress.**[3] He also identified three stages in the process of responding to stress, with different possible outcomes. The first stage is alarm, then adaptation or coping, then either resolution or exhaustion. We'll discuss this more later.

The stress response starts in the part of the brain between the brainstem and the cerebral cortex called the **limbic system,** and it is here that we interpret sensory input and initiate a responsive action. Is this incoming message a sign of danger or not? The limbic system is said to be the brain's emotional center, and it includes the **thalamus** (where sensory input is first sorted), the **amygdala** (our alarm system), and the **hippocampus** (our memory storage bank). The hippocampus compares the current moment to our past experiences in order to decide on the response we should take. (Note: there are other components of the limbic system, some of which I'll mention later, and neuroscientists don't always agree on what goes on the list.)

When we are faced with a challenge, either real or imagined, the alarm goes off in our amygdala. The body goes into red alert—a major activation of the sympathetic nervous system. Relatively minor daily threats might include preparing for an important meeting, trying to find your lost wallet, or worrying about a difficult situation that you have to deal with today. Or there could be a bigger threat to your safety, such as an oncoming vehicle in the road or another person about to attack you. Your **hypothalamus** (another part of the limbic system) instantaneously sends signals to the **adrenal glands** (a crucial part of both the nervous system and the endocrine system, in the middle of your body just above your kidneys), where hormones kick in to get you ready to meet the threat.[4] One of those hormones is **epinephrine,** also known as adrenaline. Another one is **cortisol,** one of the glucocorticoid hormones. Epi-nephrine/adrenaline works in seconds to speed us up; cortisol kicks in more slowly over minutes or hours to return the body to **homeostasis.**[5] With the adrenaline surge, blood flow is diverted from digestion and the skin to the skeletal muscles to supply extra fuel so you can act quickly and efficiently. Your heart rate and breathing rate increase to supply extra oxygen, passage-ways in the lungs dilate, and your mind shifts into a high alert state with the pupils of the eyes dilated.

Once triggered, the stress response lasts about twenty to thirty minutes, as long as the stimulus is not repeated. However, the perception of stress can last much longer, causing harmful chronic stress to the body and mind. Robert Sapolsky states in his book *Why Zebras Don't Get Ulcers* that the stress response itself, especially if it is chronic and intense, is a detriment to health in many ways. Our stress response system gets used to being stimulated and for-gets how to turn off.[6] Excessive cortisol from long-term stress is correlated with cardiovascular disease, immune deficiency, poor tissue repair, sleep problems, impaired learning, mood disorders, and endocrine imbalances, just to name a few. One of the great gifts of bodymind practice is to provide balance to this chronic stress by enhancing our "rest, digest, and repair" states of being, which are the domain of the parasympathetic nervous system.

When we are exposed to threats over a long period of time, bodymind conditioning develops; the amygdala becomes habituated to a state of ongo-ing vigilance and anticipatory fear. This in turn conditions the muscles and fascia to be in a state of constant readiness and constant tension. To some degree, we all carry this kind of tension, preset from conditioning throughout our lives. The question is: Does it limit our freedom and our well-being? And what can we do to reset our nervous system toward more ease? Stay tuned.

The main function of the **parasympathetic nervous system** is to calm the bodymind after the stress of a sympathetic stimulus, to bring us back to homeostasis. All the changes noted above are reversed: the heart rate and breathing rate slow down, blood supply to the digestive organs increases, brain activity slows down, and the eyes relax.

The **vagus nerve,** one of the cranial nerves exiting the spinal cord near the base of the skull, contains a full 80 percent of all the parasympathetic nerve fibers in the body.[7] Its name means "wanderer," reflecting its winding pathway through many of our vital organs. New research on the vagus nerve promises to provide many new approaches to stress-related conditions such as heart disease, arthritis, and depression.

Vagal tone is the ability of the vagus nerve to regulate key processes in the body toward lower excitation. When the vagus nerve is stimulated by the hypothalamus to evoke a parasympathetic response, it will slow the heart rate and dilate the blood vessels. Gentle pressure on the eyes and their surrounding bones, as when using an eye pillow in restorative yoga poses, will elicit a parasympathetic response and increase overall relaxation.

I postulate that the sustained pressure of the balls, especially at the base of the skull, could help to switch the nervous system from stress to relaxation, strengthening vagal tone. Herbert Benson, a physician and the author of several books on wellness through effective stress management,[8] popularized the notion that we can learn methods to make this switch as part of our normal daily skill set. Research is ongoing regarding the effect of vagal tone on inflammatory conditions, mood regulation, and social behaviors.

YOUR BREATH AS REGULATOR

Remember that the second kosha is the breath? The way we breathe affects the nervous system very directly. Each time you inhale, there's a small stimulus to your sympathetic nervous system, and your heart rate speeds up a little. Each time you exhale, your heart rate slows down and your body shifts toward relaxation. This is called **respiratory sinus arrhythmia.** In addition, the upper lungs have more nerve receptors for the sympathetic nervous system, whereas the lower lungs have more receptors for the parasympathetic nervous system. Fast, shallow breathing speeds you up, and slower, deeper breathing slows you down, because when we inhale deeply, we reach those parasympathetic receptors. This is one reason why bodymind modalities emphasize the conscious practice of breathing deeply and slowly to focus and calm the mind. When the breath is steady and full, the mind and body become more calm and steady as well.

NAVIGATING THE STRESS-RELAXATION SPECTRUM: CHALLENGE VERSUS THREAT

As mentioned above, we constantly fluctuate between sympathetic and parasympathetic dominance. With too much sympathetic dominance, we may be chronically agitated and then exhausted, whereas too much parasympathetic dominance can lead to lethargy and depression. Both external situations and internal thought patterns can trigger these responses; they can persist over time or change rapidly from moment to moment. The stress of jumping out of the way of an oncoming car can be physiologically the same as the stress of an intense argument, or the stress of attempting a challenging yoga pose, or the stress of anticipating anything that we fear. The difference is in our ability to distinguish between the excitement of a challenge and the fear of an injury.

Stress is beneficial and conducive to growth in appropriate doses (Hans Selye's "eustress"). If we can shift cognitively to meet a challenge without seeing it as a threat (when appropriate, of course), the body responds with the quick-acting epinephrine, but without the overdose of cortisol.[9] Here is one of the many delicate interactions between our thoughts and our physiology, inviting us to examine how we perceive our world and how that perception affects our health.

The sympathetic response is all or nothing (when stimulated, everything goes into red alert), but the parasympathetic system can be activated one portion at a time and has many "switches."[10] In Bodymind Ballwork, the steady pressure of the ball, the steady flow of the breath, and slow and steady movement all contribute to an overall composite switch toward parasympathetic dominance. And I have found that this effect gets stronger with practice.

CONDITIONS FOR RELAXATION

Here are some other ways to enhance relaxation when you are practicing the ballwork:

1. Reduce internal stimuli (for example, avoid caffeine).

2. Time your practice for best results. Notice your stress patterns through-out your day, and practice when you most need it.

3. Limit your sensory input, which means being comfortably cool or warm, and having a relatively quiet environment.

4. Consciously let go of muscular tension as much as you can.

5. Breathe deeply and slowly.

6. Concentrate on what you are doing, noticing your physical sensations, and gently guiding your mind away from worries, plans, fears, memories, etc.

7. Practice regularly. Your bodymind will gradually retrain itself toward intentional relaxation when you need it. You'll become conditioned to let go of mental and physical tension when you feel the balls against your body.

In the next chapter, we'll look more closely at the connective tissue of the body, how pain is registered in the body, and how relaxation occurs from the pressure of the balls.

CHAPTER 3

Soft Tissues, Pain, and Release

Let's look more closely at the tissues that come in contact with the balls when you do Bodymind Ballwork, and how they respond. The four primary types of tissue in the body are epithelial, muscle, nerve, and connective tissue.

Epithelial tissue includes the skin, the linings of organs, and the glands. There are pressure receptors in the skin that receive stimuli by touch. The response to that stimuli varies, as we'll discuss below.

Muscle tissue, whose main job is to contract, produces movement. There are three types of muscles: striated or skeletal muscles, which move the joints; smooth or visceral muscles, which move the organs; and cardiac muscles, which pump the heart. When we work with the balls, we are creating pressure in the skeletal muscles nearest to the surface of the body, and indirectly to the visceral muscles when we work on the abdomen. This pressure can result in a softening of contractions held in the muscle, and an increase in circulation of blood and interstitial fluids.

Nerve tissue carries electrochemical messages between the brain and every part of the body at a miraculous speed (see chart in chapter 2). The motor and sensory nerves of the peripheral nervous system are located throughout the body, some closer to the surface and others deeper, from head to toes and fingers. Each nerve has a protective coating of three layers of connective tissue. As we each can attest, some parts of the body are more richly supplied with nerves than others; we feel with much more detail and can do more detailed movements with our fingers as compared with our elbows or knees. It's not harmful to create pressure on the nerves with the balls, but of course it's best to use common sense and avoid pressure where there is extreme sensitivity.

Connective tissue is the most abundant type of tissue in the body, and the most varied in its texture, shape, and function. Some types of connective tissue are liquid, such as blood and lymph. Others are soft padding materials such as areolar tissue and adipose tissue (also known as fat), and harder padding tissues like cartilage. Bones are classified as connective tissue, and due to their high mineral content, bones are solid enough to provide support (in our spine, arms, and legs) and protection (in our skull). There are also many types of semi-pliable connective tissues such as ligaments (bone to bone), tendons (muscle to bone), and fascia, the all-pervasive connector whose functions are essential for coordinating our movements.[1]

FASCIA

Fascia is our organizing matrix, the biological web that serves to both connect and separate virtually every structure in the body. It provides cushioning just under the skin; it wraps around and through every muscle (here called myofascia); it supports the bones, the organs, and even the blood vessels and nerves. The texture of fascia can be thin or thick, gel-like or more solid, depending on its local function. It provides our internal structure to a large extent, and it is richly supplied with sensory nerves. Research into the characteristics and functions of fascia has gathered momentum over recent years, with insights that relate to all forms of movement education and healing.[2]

TENSEGRITY

Once we recognize the pervasiveness and continuity of the fascial web, we see that our body structure is not just dependent on the bones, the joints, and the muscles that move them. It is a dynamic structure in which the bones float in a continuous, supportive, and mobile web of soft tissue. Because that web provides both stretchability (meaning it is tensile) and integrity (it gives support), Buckminster Fuller coined a term for this: **tensegrity.** In a tensegrity structure, none of the solid elements actually touch each other, but they are separated and supported by the softer tensile elements. The term "biotensegrity" is used to specify the tensegrity structure of the human body.

We often attribute aches and pains to muscles, but with knowledge of the fascial web, we see that body problems are rarely caused by a single muscle's dysfunction. Every movement pulls on the fascial web that spans the body in different patterns of connectivity. This is force transmission, happening 24/7. Without force transmission, we wouldn't be able to push off for a jump or skillfully swing a tennis racket while on the run. The fascia is constantly participating in and responding to whatever movements we do. Because fascia constitutes 30 percent of a muscle's bulk and it creates the interface with neighboring structures, the consistency of our fascia can be a significant factor in our overall flexibility and our susceptibility to injury.

Even though it may appear to be quite thick and tough, fascia is largely composed of water. It is made of an extracellular matrix, plus various types of cells. The extracellular matrix is made of 90 percent water, plus fibers such as collagen, elastin, and reticulin. Collagen provides structural support and tensile strength, and elastin provides (not surprisingly) elasticity. The fluid part, also known as ground substance, is where all chemical exchanges take place; nutrients are being absorbed and waste products are being removed. This fluid can be watery, allowing easier movement, or more viscous (like syrup), with more resistance to movement. Good hydration makes the fascia spongier and more resilient, but drinking lots of water while staying on the couch doesn't do the trick! We hydrate the tissues only when we move the body enough to circulate the fluids. Also, when the fascia is warmed internally by movement or externally by heat, its viscosity is lowered, making movement easier. We postulate that manual therapies, exercise, and ballwork can lower the viscosity of the ground substance (i.e., "melt" it) and facilitate movement of fluids through the fascia. With good hydration and nutrition, the tissues can remain flexible and repair themselves as needed. Practitioners of ballwork often use words like "liquid" or "fluid" when describing the feeling inside their body after using the balls.

Fascia contains many different types of collagen, which vary in their flexibility and other properties. We are each born with a certain blend of these types of collagen. Even though our alignment and movements do make a huge difference in our flexibility, our heredity (and probably nutrition as well) will affect how easily we can bend, move, and stretch. Besides heredity and activity level, age is also a factor; our collagen degrades as we age.

Although we cannot contract our fascia consciously, as we can contract muscles, recent research has found that smooth muscle cells within the myofascia respond to stress by contracting.[3] It doesn't matter whether the stress is psychological, chemical, or structural. The body automatically braces to try to support itself, and the fascial tissue tightens in response.

Let's take an example of structural stress that is very common. Perhaps you hold your hips to the right side for a prolonged period of time, due to your daily habits or some other cause, like scoliosis in your spine. The fascia and muscles on the sides of your hips and lower back will become thicker and tighter on the left, attempting to support the weight of your upper body without the help of the pelvis being centered under them. Even though the muscles are in a stretched position, they remain in a state of chronic contraction that anatomist Thomas Myers calls "locked long" (known in physiotherapy as eccentrically loaded). Conversely, the fascia and muscles on the other side will be "locked short" (or concentrically loaded).[4] Both sides are essentially weak—one because it's too busy holding things together, and the other side because it's inactive. The discomfort will probably be felt in the long side, but without opening the short side, we won't find balance. Stretching the achy long side will only worsen the problem.

What if your daily life involves very little movement, or movement in only a few directions or in only a small range, even if that movement is vigorous? In my parents' generation, many people assumed that just going through your day (with an occasional sports activity) was enough exercise to stay healthy, and until fairly recently the characteristics of fascia were not well known. We now know that when fascia is not regularly stimulated by varied and full-range movements, its layers can get stuck together, creating adhesions almost like random packing tape inside the body. When the various layers of fascia don't glide over each other smoothly, the result can be areas of thickened tissue, movement restriction, inflammation, and eventually pain.[5] You might say, "As I get older, I'm getting stiffer, less coordinated, more stooped in my posture, and I have chronic back pain, and it's all part of normal aging." That may be true, but now we know that intelligent, varied movement and specific therapeutic interventions can lessen these seemingly inevitable changes. And much of it happens in the fascia.

What does all this mean for the practice of Bodymind Ballwork? The balls give an entry point to change the patterns of tension in the fascial web. They give pressure at various angles to both muscle tissue and fascia, bringing greater fluid circulation and gradually breaking up adhesions (layers of tissues glued together) and easing muscle contractions. Receptors within our soft tissues signal a change toward relaxation, reflexes causing contraction are interrupted, and the tissue gradually opens up and releases. Once the fascia is more resilient and movable, our movements become more easeful and we have more choice about how to align ourselves.

Joyce, an actress, says, "I wake up almost every morning with back pain, probably due to the asymmetries on my spine. When I use the balls, it relieves tension and pressure in the painful spots. I'm getting more and more skilled at choosing what balls to use, where to place them, and how long to remain on them. It has really helped me."

PAIN, RECEPTORS, AND RESPONSES

New students often ask me this question when they first feel the ball's pressure: "Is this ballwork supposed to hurt?" The answer is no; causing pain is certainly not the purpose of the work. But there is often discomfort when we begin to practice if we have carried chronic tension for a long time. Healthy skeletal muscles are designed to contract and release as needed to move our bones, but often they "forget" how to release. When the muscles are contracted over long periods of time, metabolic waste products build up, activating sensory nerve receptors. There are **chemoreceptors** (detecting chemical changes), **mechanoreceptors** (detecting mechanical pressure), and **nociceptors** (detecting pain). Each kind of receptor elicits a slightly different kind of pain: chemoreceptors cause burning, aching, or fatigue; mechanoreceptors can cause cramping; and nociceptors cause feelings of pinching, stabbing, or tearing.[6] These sensations can originate in muscle tissue, but perhaps even more so in the fascia surrounding the muscles.

Pressure against the soft tissue, with a massage therapist's hand or a tool such as a ball, will evoke a response from the mechanoreceptors. There are several kinds of mechanoreceptors, each with its own specialties. **Golgi tendon organs** register the degree of tension in a muscle/tendon structure, and if there is a danger of tearing, these mechanoreceptors signal the muscle to release. **Pacinian corpuscles** respond to rapidly changing stimuli, and help the tissue prepare for activity. **Interstitial receptors,** also known as free nerve endings, are the most abundant type, found everywhere from skin to bone. They supply the feedback we need for proprioception, knowing where our body parts are and how we are moving. They respond to light touch, but also to the kind of shearing deeper pressure that comes from massage and ballwork.

The mechanoreceptor that is responsive to slow pressure is the **Ruffini corpuscle** (also known as the Ruffini ending). It is found on the ends of certain sensory nerves near the skin, and in deeper soft tissues of the body such as fascia, ligaments, and joint capsules. Angelo Ruffini was an Italian anatomist who named and described these structures in 1898. When Ruffini corpuscles are stimulated by sustained pressure against the skin, and into the underlying fascia, they signal the autonomic nervous system to switch from sympathetic to parasympathetic dominance—in other words, relaxation.[7] This explains the effect of general relaxation that occurs while practicing Bodymind Ballwork, regardless of which part of the body you are working with. For example, people often describe a sense of overall calm when they have worked on just one body part. Carol, a mother of three, says that she can switch gears after a hectic day with just a few minutes of ballwork on her shoulders and neck.

PAIN IS SUBJECTIVE

Sometimes the ballwork brings chronic pain to the surface; it was there all along, but we have become numb to it over time. Physical pain is subjective; we each have our own tolerance level and ways of dealing with it. Acute pain from a traumatic injury or surgery makes itself known without subtlety and can be unrelenting. But often we carry chronic pain in the body that's just under the surface, perhaps not consciously acknowledged. We become so accustomed to it that we no longer feel it, but it affects our behavior. Have you noticed that chronic pain can make you less patient or less able to concentrate? When we have chronic pain, we also might choose to avoid moving that part of the body, for fear that the pain will increase. This numbing effect further reduces our movement range and our freedom of expression.

When we are under stress, our nervous system activates into a state of vigilance, ready to act. Muscles are on alert, in partial and constant contraction. Cells called **myofibroblasts** within the fascia have the capacity to contract when stimulated by the chemicals of stress or the need for repair, as in closing a wound. Some scenarios that might apply here are: You are at your computer, working toward a deadline, not able to take time to stretch, and your shoulders, arms, and neck muscles stay in a permanent state of contraction. Or you are in a family or social situation that poses danger to you—embarrassment, injury, abuse, or rejection—and your body cringes into a protective stance that becomes a habit. The fascia becomes tight and restricts your freedom of movement and your proprioception. An extreme example of this is post-traumatic stress disorder, discussed in chapter 5, when the bodymind internalizes psychological trauma, which then becomes locked in the tissues. We may need some intervention to interrupt the myofascial tension and gradually help it to return to a healthier state. And that intervention might not be comfortable at first.

OUTGOING AND INCOMING PAIN

While working with the balls, it's useful to distinguish between what I call "outgoing" and "incoming" pain. We feel "outgoing" pain when the balls contact a part of the body that is chronically contracted from overwork or protection, but that is hopefully ready to release. The pressure does not cause the pain, but reveals it. A common example of this is pain in the shoulder muscles as the ball starts to dig into a tight trapezius muscle after too much time at the computer. Outgoing pain hurts, but we have the instinctual feeling that it's a "good" pain and ready to shift.

"Incoming" pain is pain that is caused by an external stimulus, such as the pain of disturbing a wound that is healing. If you have a recent injury, your tissues might still be inflamed, and the ball can cause incoming pain. In this case it's best to change to a softer ball or avoid the most intense places until some improvement has occurred by other means.

As you practice the ballwork over long periods of time, you can monitor your levels of discomfort or pain in different parts of your body and watch for changes. You can use the pain scale of 1-10: 1 is slight discomfort, 10 is extreme pain. For instance, you might work on your trapezius for the first time and rate the pain level at 7 or 8, but after a few sessions, it might be down to a 4 or 5. It's a useful way to track your progress.

Once we come to be aware of pain and tension, we can ask ourselves: Why is this tension there? What function does it have for me? Is it compensating for poor alignment? Is it a movement pattern that is stuck in the "on" position and can't let go because of overwork? Is it connected to fear or some other emotional state? Do I want to know more about it?

This kind of self-reflection is an essential part of a bodymind practice. In the next chapter, we'll look at how we create an internalized picture of our body and our self as a whole. That picture is called the body schema.

CHAPTER 4

Body Schema, Body Image, and Conditioning

How do you know who you are and where you are? Do you define yourself with your age, your looks, your job, your dreams, your relationships? Do your body sensations factor into your identity? From the time we are in the womb, we develop a sense of our own individual body and all of its parts, which we call the **body schema.** It's a felt sense of the body parts, how they fit together and how they relate to the environment around us, including other people. We know the general size and shape of our body, its boundaries, and that it is ours and not someone else's. We feel the pull of gravity, knowing that the ground is under us. Our body schema includes **proprioception** (feeling our posture and the body moving) and **interoception** (feeling inner sensations such as our heart rate, heat and cold, thirst and hunger, digestion, pain and pleasure, sensuality). We also have a personal picture of what our body looks like to others—not necessarily an accurate one—and this is called our **body image.** But how do we know this?

Paul Schilder, in his book *The Image and Appearance of the Human Body*, writes:

> We do not know very much about our body unless we move it. Movement is a great unifying factor between the different parts of our body. By movement we come into a definitive relationship to the

outside world and to objects, and only in contact with this outside world are we able to correlate the diverse impressions concerning our own body.[1]

Our body schema and body image are dynamic, always affected by experiences and changing throughout life. Adolescents typically go through intense fluctuations in their body image, as societal pressures, physical changes, and hormones put the pressure on. Perhaps the way you thought of yourself as an adolescent is different from the way you see yourself now. Perhaps even now as an adult, you have external pressures that cause you to judge your body for its appearance. For those whose body image has become largely negative, some intervention can help to redefine and relearn oneself in an authentic self-supporting way. This intervention can be a combination of psychotherapy and bodywork. Self-awareness—both conceptual and embodied—needs constant renewal. The promise of bodywork is to help us to update and refine our body schema and body image as we go through life. We gain a deeper and more nuanced self-awareness of who we are, and more capacity for self-regulation and self-acceptance.

TOUCH AND BODY SCHEMA

The body schema begins to form in the womb. After birth, infants learn about their world through touching, exploring everything around them with mouths and fingers and toes. Touch is food for the nervous system; we learn from it and get feedback about ourselves and our boundaries through touch. This strong influence of touch continues throughout life, often unconsciously, as we interact with our world. As part of your day, you probably handle tools and objects that blend with and extend your body schema. If you drive a vehicle, use a computer mouse or a tennis racket, play a musical instrument, or stir a soup, you are extending your body to include an object, and thereby extending your body schema into action. You learn intuitively from that interaction. Like these other helpful objects, the balls become a part of your body schema as you work with them. You can use them to learn about your body in a unique and very effective way.

Human touch is rich in emotional communication, and how we experience touch emotionally can vary tremendously. When infants are handled lovingly and their nervous systems learn to trust the touch of others, the pattern is set for touch to be a pleasurable and soothing part of their physical experience throughout life. Loving parental touch and gentle physical guidance as the child learns basic motor skills like rolling over, sitting up, and walking help to build a positive body schema for the child. But for those children whose early experiences of touch are threatening, painful, or nonexistent, physical touch becomes frightening and something to be avoided. One result of this early fear is for the body to armor itself and carry tremendous muscle tension as a protection. Shoulders stiffen, the spine stiffens, and interoception is gradually eroded. When this armoring continues for years, a person's body schema is diminished, and the bodily experiences that might offer joy and satisfaction become dangers instead.[2]

Manual therapy in a professional and safe setting can gradually help to rebuild a healthy body schema. Massage therapy is a valuable modality that has not yet taken its rightful place in the modern health care system. But if massage seems threatening, or feels like an invasion of privacy, or is not available, working with the balls can be a good first step in relearning to enjoy touch. You can choose balls that feel safe and appealing, not intrusive or threatening. The balls are nonpersonal, nonsexual, and playful, providing a touch interaction that can help rebuild a healthy body schema, and with this a sense of living more fully in the body, knowing its boundaries and its pleasures.

Dianne, an artist, had pain in her neck for so long that she became fearful of any intervention or contact with that part of her body. She held it stiffly, which compounded the problem. Gradually she learned to trust the ball as something she could control, and use to help herself. On days when her neck was particularly sore, she'd choose a very soft ball for a gentle intervention. On better days, she could address the tension with a firmer ball. She says, "One big problem with injuries is that you start to feel antagonistic toward your body. Doing the ballwork changes your relationship with your problem area because you find that you can work with it gently, and good changes happen."

POSTURE

What kind of instruction did you get as a child about posture? When I was growing up, we were just told to "stand up straight," but never told what that really meant. It seemed stiff and arbitrary to me. In my adult life as an avid mover, dancer, and yoga teacher, I have expanded my understanding of "good posture" to include much more than the static military posture implied as the goal when I was young. To me, good posture is aligning myself in the best biomechanical and expressive way for whatever I am doing. It's hardly ever "straight," but it is "up" and it is dynamic, not static. Gravity pulls us down; our challenge as two-legged creatures is to lift ourselves up and avoid the tendency to collapse. Strength is required, but it's not brute strength. An inner expansion, which goes along with a deep breath, is the best way to start to lift the spine out of a slump. When I work with students who say they want to improve their posture, we usually start with the breath, and with a suggestion of opening from the inside.

Once that inner expansion has started to happen, the next step is to soften patterns of outer tension that pull us down. If you sit at a desk all day, the muscles and fascia on the front of your body will shorten, pulling the spine into a rounded shape. The back muscles then adapt to that shape and tighten in response, so you have tension in both the back and the front. You can stretch and attempt to reverse the pattern, but only with extreme effort. Ballwork can gradually release the shortened and stiff muscles and fascia, so that achieving a taller, more open posture is not only possible, but easy and natural. Once the soft tissue is more even on the front and the back, you can do yoga or conventional exercise to strengthen the necessary supporting muscles to maintain the new posture.

As mentioned in the previous chapter, the fascia in the body is connected from top to bottom, back to front, and side to side. Changing our posture might not be as simple as pulling our shoulders back. We may need to address hidden tight areas in several parts of the body that are causing a restriction in the fascia. The balls provide an entry point into the web, a way to begin. As one part releases, we follow the web to gradually and sequentially release enough so that standing tall is effortless.

Morrie is a professional musician whose spine is kyphotic, which means that her upper back is rounded and her shoulders curve forward. She also has osteoporosis, a condition of low bone density with increased risk of fracture. Posture is important for Morrie, both to get a good breath for playing her clarinet, and to avoid a vertebral fracture. She finds that the ballwork and yoga have helped her improve her posture, and she has greatly reduced pain in her neck and shoulders. She says, "I feel stronger and I'm much more aware of my posture."

Research shows that postural patterns can affect and possibly even create our mental state. Experimental subjects who were instructed to maintain postures of collapse or protectiveness reported feelings of depression and stress.[3] Our moods and our posture, or more broadly our body carriage, are interwoven in a dynamic system that is open to change from either direction. The cycle might go like this: If we are feeling happy, the body is energized, and movements are smooth and easeful, which in turn supports our light-hearted mood. On another day, we may feel depressed or scared. Then the body goes into a protective mode: our muscles tighten, our posture becomes distorted, and that physical restriction becomes an expression of our mood while also perpetuating it. The mind and the body are in a constant dialogue and dance. Body awareness practices like Bodymind Ballwork can help us to navigate these mood and posture interactions more skillfully. Feeling anxious? Check in with your body and breath. Feeling stiff or achy? Check in with your body, your breath, and your inner voice.

THE INNER DIALOGUE

One way to check in with our interoception—our inner sense of subjective presence in the body—is with an inner dialogue, also called our internalized voice. Think for a moment about whether you have an inner dialogue, a way of checking in with yourself throughout your day. If you do, what are its contours and themes? Do you talk to yourself with judgment, criticism, or disapproval? Or are you an encouraging coach for yourself? Does your body have a voice in the conversation? Do you find fault with your body, or berate it for giving you pain? Do you ruminate about the causes of body problems? Do you compare your body with other people's bodies? Do you listen to what your body has to tell you? If you are feeling tired or irritable, does your body have a message for you? If your neck hurts and you are short-tempered, can you see the connection between those two states? Do you see your body as an ally, or an adversary? A burden, or your very own self?

I believe that we develop our inner dialogue over our lifetime. It is influenced by our family and by the culture we live in, the education we receive, the work that we do, and our goals for ourselves. I often ask students what they were taught about self-care while growing up. For many of us, it's the usual short list: eat healthy food, get exercise, get enough sleep. Rarely is anything taught about the value of interoception or embodied self-awareness—the ongoing process of dialogue between your mental and physical selves. Without an authentic subjective connection with ourselves, the conglomeration of stresses that life brings takes a bigger toll.

Of course, this inner dialogue is colored by memories, both conscious ones and unconscious ones. Many of the writers I refer to in this book have described these two kinds of memories, calling them explicit memories and implicit memories.[4] **Explicit memories** have to do with autobiographical, narrative, and factual details (where you grew up, what you did for vacation last year, how to cook an egg). These memories are strengthened by repetition and can help us navigate the practical aspects of life. Parenting books advocate talking to children about the sequence of daily events in their lives as a way to increase their ability to sequence their thoughts and create a context for memories that will help them learn.[5]

Implicit memories are those from sensory and emotional experiences that we may not consciously recall but that leave an imprint. We store implicit memories throughout our lives, but especially in the first eighteen to twenty-four months, when that is the only kind of memory being formed.[6] Examples include knowing the faces of family members, recognizing the smell of a favorite food, or being scared of the power of ocean waves. Other examples involving personal interactions might be the feeling of shame when scolded by a stern teacher, or the feeling of love and trust when cared for by a loving parent. These memories form the substratum for our sense of who we are and how the world works. That doesn't mean that they define us—we have agency for re-creating ourselves in every moment—but that we carry these implicit memories that could influence our current experiences.

CONDITIONING AND SAMSKARAS

In yoga, implicit memories are referred to as samskaras. **Samskaras** are the imprints from our previous experiences that affect our current life in the form of beliefs, habits, and tendencies. They run the gamut from positive to neutral to negative. What's an example of a samskara? Some might call it an instinct or a desire, like always wanting to eat a sweet dessert after a meal. Another example is a mental/emotional pattern, like distrust of lawyers or doctors because of a previous bad experience, or the tendency to romantically bond with a certain type of person. Samskaras can also show up as our physical habits. Perhaps a lifetime of playing basketball leaves a positive imprint of pleasure in quick, light movements. A life spent doing hard physical labor leaves the imprint of tremendous muscular strength but also tremendous fatigue. Years of sitting still at work might leave an imprint of immobility that comes to be the norm. In each case, a repeated physical state or movement becomes a habit, which then become our posture and movement style, which then become our biological and mental structure, and the cycle begins again.

In 1998, child development professionals coined the term "adverse childhood experiences," or ACEs.[7] The theory states that difficult circumstances in childhood create deep-seated changes that carry through a person's life, long after the stressful situation has outwardly ended. The stress might be a one-time event, such as the death of a parent, or it might be constant and long-lasting, such as an abusive or mentally ill parent, physical illness, or extreme poverty.

When a child faces chronic and unpredictable stressors, their developing body and brain become routinely flooded with inflammatory stress chemicals. This flood alters the expression of genes that control stress hormone output, triggering an overactive inflammatory stress response for life. When these changes occur in genes that should regulate a healthy stress response, a child's inflammatory stress response becomes permanently set to "on"—and the homeostatic mechanisms that should turn off that stress response don't work. These **epigenetic**[8] changes can predispose an individual to lifelong inflammation and propensity for many adult diseases. There is also evidence that the epigenetic changes like these can be carried over from one generation to another. In one experiment, for instance, mice were exposed to a stressor and a simultaneous smell of cherry blossoms. Future generations from those mice had abnormal stress responses to the same smell without exposure to the stressor. What your grandmother had to deal with in her lifetime may still be resonating in your consciousness!

When you work slowly and mindfully to explore your body sensations and movement with Bodymind Ballwork, you will gradually build an understanding of how conditioning and implicit memories have created your body schema of today. With repeated practice, you come to trust the safety of the balls and the inner journey that is opened up by embodied self-awareness, and you can make changes. Emotions and implicit memories lodged in the tissues of the body begin to dissolve, with or without making themselves known to your conscious mind. Experiences of the past may bubble up unexpectedly, offering you the opportunity to know yourself more deeply. You may find that you have the choice to let go of some of the conditioning that holds you back from your full expression. But if there are complex factors that disconnect you from your body, reconnecting might seem too risky. In the next chapter, we'll outline some ways in which interoception and the development of a healthy body schema may be hijacked.

CHAPTER 5

Defense Mechanisms and Trauma

Thus far our emphasis has been on the health benefits of improving interoception, giving oneself opportunities and support for an internal self-awareness. But there are situations in which interoception can feel dangerous and like something to be avoided. In the situations described here, the connection between mind and body becomes skewed and takes us away from being present in embodied self-awareness. We defend ourselves from outer threats—either real or imagined—but also threats from inside ourselves. Note that each one of these defenses can manifest in degrees, from mild to moderate to extreme, and they are difficult to objectively measure.

Repression is the process of burying a feeling that is intolerable, and making it invisible to the conscious mind. Whether it is a childhood trauma, an unwelcome pattern of thoughts, or a forbidden desire, we may need to repress the feeling in order to go on with life. Residues of the repressed emotion can lodge in the body and may surface at any time without warning. Repressed feelings might cause muscular pain or stiffness, as the body takes on what the mind rejects. We hold ourselves back from the feeling by literally holding tension in the tissues.

In the defense called **sublimation** we transform socially or personally unacceptable emotional urges into other, more acceptable expressions. Whereas some might say that this is a positive process of maturation, others might argue that it compromises our emotional expression and therefore also our embodied self-awareness. Sublimation serves a purpose but comes with a cost if our true but unexpressed emotion lodges in the body as physical tension or pain.

Detachment occurs when we are unable to stay connected to the sensations of our body (or some part of it) because of fear or avoidance of discomfort. To some degree, this is a natural response to pain: we move away from pain, and therefore we move away from including the body in our sense of self. It becomes a problem when it is so habitual that we are disconnected from our body most of the time. Embodied self-awareness is not always easy, and involves tolerating ambiguity and discomfort, but in the long run, it's worthwhile.

Somatization is the exaggeration of self-awareness, in which we become fixated on a physical symptom and attach more significance to it than is necessary or appropriate. Benign sensations become causes for alarm, and the nervous system rallies its immune response where none is needed. The energy drain of stress from somatization can itself cause symptoms of illness such as muscle weakness, depression, and fatigue.

Intellectualization is an attempt to turn away from embodied feelings by interpreting, judging, and overanalyzing a physical symptom. Given the nature of our current medical system, it is easy to go for test after test, and to rely on the expertise of others to assess what's going on in our body, to the exclusion of feeling and accepting our sensations. Contemplative work such as Bodymind Ballwork gives an immediate and subjective experience of the "here and now" in the body, undercutting the tendency to intellectualize bodily experience.

Compartmentalization is the process of separating out emotional aspects of an experience while dealing with a challenge. It can be expressed as "deal but don't feel."[1] In practical terms, this might be necessary if facing an emergency. We don't need to feel the actions or responses of our bodies consciously while we run for safety during an earthquake. But if that habit of not feeling persists, we may lose the capacity to be subjectively present, which robs us of part of our innate body intelligence.

When we are stuck in **rumination,** we replay negative patterns of thoughts, fears, and regrets so often that we lose the capacity to feel ourselves in the present moment. The mind takes over with repeating patterns of negativities that are self-sustaining and keep us from embodied self-awareness or active problem solving. Working with the balls helps to bring us to the present moment—to ask, What exactly is going on in my body right now?

Addiction is a strong subjective desire for a certain substance or activity, with disregard for any possible negative physiological or social consequences. One can be addicted to alcohol, recreational drugs, pharmaceutical drugs, caffeine, sugar, sex, watching television, playing video games, gambling, extreme exercise regimes, etc. Pleasure seeking overtakes any rational decision making, and the addict feels unable to restrain the urge to obtain the desired substance or do the desired activity. **Dopamine** is a neurotransmitter produced in the brainstem; its normal function is to motivate us to seek pleasure. In addiction, the brain circuits for self-regulation of cravings are working abnormally, and urges for the "high" from the desired substance or activity go unchecked by higher cognitive processes. One way to subvert addiction is to gradually develop habits of self-care that are pleasurable and not harmful, such as the pleasure of releasing tight muscles and fascia. Health-promoting practices can also become addictive in a positive way.

Post-traumatic stress disorder is an extreme example of disturbance of the body schema and interoception. When a person witnesses or is part of a severely upsetting event (like 9/11, a war experience, a violent criminal act, a natural disaster, or childhood abuse), the stress response can take various forms, encapsulated by the "fight, flight, or freeze" triad. Often the event causes a need for some strong action that has to be repressed or cannot be completed: either screaming, fighting back, running away, or somehow preventing harm to oneself or others. The unexpressed energy of that thwarted action becomes embedded in the bodymind and remains deep inside, ready to burst out when triggered. A trigger can be anything that reminds the person of the trauma—a sight, smell, sound, body position, object, etc.

Symptoms of PTSD include a persistently high state of arousal, intrusive memories and flashbacks, difficulty concentrating, avoidance of circumstances that may evoke memories, negative changes in mood, and emotional reactions like extreme anxiety, guilt, or anger. People may also settle into a state of hypo-arousal—a kind of lethargy and hopelessness. Body schema is impaired, and there is a detachment from the body as a reliable source of comfort. In the brain there is hyperactivity in the amygdala and insula, with loss of ability to regulate the fear response cognitively in the cerebral cortex. Memories become lodged in the tissues, remaining for years or reemerging when triggered.[2]

Bessel van der Kolk, a leading researcher and expert on trauma, has many valuable insights to offer. In describing the huge challenges faced by survivors, he says:

> Despite the human capacity to survive and adapt, traumatic experiences can alter people's psychological, biological, and social equilibrium to such a degree that memory (conscious or unconscious) of one particular event comes to taint all other experiences, spoiling appreciation of the present. The tyranny of the past interferes with the ability to pay attention to both new and familiar situations.... Life tends to become colorless, and contemporary experience ceases to be a teacher.[3]

Children who suffer abuse or neglect by their primary caregivers are likely to dissociate from their body as an escape mechanism. This abuse can take a range of forms: lack of basic care, lack of love, physical or psychological abuse, or sexual violation. Body schema and bodymind boundaries have been violated at an age when there are few internal resources, and patterns of fear, detachment, or anger can become lodged in the nervous system. Years later, when dealing with a persistent physical symptom, a victim of abuse may discover that the current symptom functions as a cover for memories that have been too painful to face. Trauma survivors might go to any length to try to make the emotional pain disappear: self-cutting, alcohol, drugs, starvation, binge eating, or numbing of the body through intense physical challenges.

Touch can be so frightening for abuse survivors that massage is out of the question. But working with the balls can provide the same soothing and relaxing effect on the muscles and fascia as massage, without the intrusion of personal touch. Whereas previous touch experiences might have brought a mixture of pleasure, pain, betrayal, and manipulation, the safe and neutral touch of the balls can help to reset the bodymind's conditioned response of fear. We can actually rewire the brain with positive experiences of physical contact.

Bessel van der Kolk says it this way:

> The challenge is: How can people gain control over the residues of past trauma and return to being masters of their own ship? Talking, understanding, and human connections help, and drugs can dampen hyperactive alarm systems. But we will also see that the imprints from the past can be transformed by having physical experiences that directly contradict the helplessness, rage, and collapse that are part of trauma, and thereby regaining self-mastery.[4]

David, a dancer and bodywork teacher, suffered abuse as a child and has found the ballwork to be an invaluable practice:

In the years that I first began to understand the consequences of the harmful experiences of my childhood, I tended to objectify and work forcefully with my body. To be attentive to my own physicality was distressing. Sometimes noticing the touch of the balls against my skin seemed like an inventory of my hurt and suffering. I tended to avoid noticing the sensations of my body by silencing them with intense dance classes, Pilates workouts, and long stints on the dance floors of underground nightclubs. The message that I existed to fulfill someone else's needs felt like it had been planted in my mind, muscles, ligaments, and connective tissue.

Working with the balls helped change how I perceived the experiences of my body. Over time, I learned how my perceptions of what was happening in my body were often quieter and kinder than my internal monologue. The therapists and support groups that were trying to help me often reiterated the terrible things I told myself about myself. Movement, sensation, and feeling were a different process. Slowly, I learned how the sensation of touch could allow me a sense of internal quiet. When I was no longer fixated on healing, I could notice the infinite complexity and subtlety of the touch and movement of the balls against my skin. Touch led to feeling; feeling led to space; space led to being; being allowed me self-acceptance and transformation. The sense of internal spaciousness I began to experience let me be gentle with my body and myself.

Not needing to repeat who I was to myself, I wondered who I might be, how I felt in the one spot where the ball was touching me at one moment. Sensation's indeterminacy began to define me more than a narrative or pathology. When I stopped demanding certainty from my experience with the balls, discomfort was no longer a catastrophe for me. Distinctions like being broken or unbroken, safe or unsafe, traumatized or normal became less important to me than the infinite varieties of my muscle tone and the subtleties of my proprioception. The playground of finding and refinding my embodiment became a safe house for my growing and changing self.

How else can bodywork help to free trauma survivors of this suffering? Let's look at the brain again to see where and how positive change can happen. Note that although we can associate specific functions with specific parts of the brain, our awareness is a "whole systems phenomenon," involving many parts simultaneously.[5]

THE CINGULATE CORTEX AND INSULAR CORTEX: CENTERS OF INTEROCEPTION AND SELF-REGULATION

How can we find the capacity to be true to our emotions, and also make smart choices about our behavior? In other words, how can we coordinate the heart and the mind? The amygdala, our alarm system, registers raw emotions that are fed by survival instincts, and the cerebral cortex (our inner executive) makes the decisions of how to respond. Daniel J. Siegel and Tina Payne Bryson, in their book *The Whole-Brain Child,* describe this dichotomy as "downstairs" and "upstairs" functioning.[6] The "downstairs" responses are rapid and intense, sensing danger and getting us ready to fight or flee. The "upstairs" responses are more measured, using cognitive processes to think through what is happening and to choose a response.[7]

Bridging the limbic system (downstairs) and the cerebral cortex (upstairs), there are two areas where we regulate our responses to the raw emotions registering in the limbic system. Both are involved with interoception, so we can safely assume that bodywork practices develop these areas of the brain.

The **cingulate cortex,** located just below the cerebral cortex and above the limbic system, has several subsections. The **anterior cingulate cortex** determines where our attention is directed. It also is the place where we mobilize our actions in relation to emotions.[8] Research shows that mindfulness meditation, involving the intention to stay in the present and notice sensations, stimulates and strengthens the anterior cingulate cortex.[9] Other areas of the cingulate cortex are also associated with movement as an expression of emotion.[10]

The **insular cortex** receives information from the thalamus about all types of sensations in the body. It sorts these sensory messages and relays them to higher areas in the cerebral cortex for the next step of action planning. The insular cortex is believed to be central to our self-awareness, our interoception, our agency in knowing our own movements, our evaluation of pain, and our ability to empathize with others.

THE PREFRONTAL CORTEX

Another stage up on the neuroaxis (the line from older, lower brain functions up to the more evolved cerebral cortex) is the **prefrontal cortex.** James Austin, author of *Zen and the Brain,* sums up its functions well:

> Prefrontal functions inject an open pause into what would otherwise be a headlong reflex pattern of stimulus-response. Into this gap, they insert some flexible behavioral options, chosen on the basis of hard-won practical experience, even reason. So the prefrontal cortex does more than keep tabs on things that happened to work—or fail—in the past. It projects fresh options into the future. And having weighed how practical and proper each act is, it keeps monitoring our ongoing behavior and fine-tuning it on a moment-to-moment basis.[11]

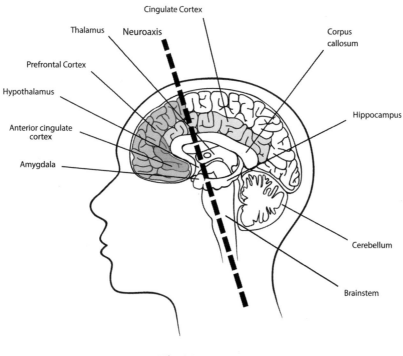

The Neuroaxis

Now we'll look at further divisions of the prefrontal cortex, because they are so relevant to embodied self-awareness. There are three to consider.

The **orbital prefrontal cortex** (OPFC) is named for its proximity to the bony orbits that contain our eyes. This is where we control impulsive urges and any socially unacceptable behaviors. It counters the amygdala's urgent alarm signal and allows for a more measured response to our surroundings.

The **dorsomedial prefrontal cortex** (DMPFC) is where we generate thoughts about ourselves. It's the seat of conceptual self-awareness, our more analytical way of understanding our moment-to-moment experience. In contrast, the **ventromedial prefrontal cortex** (VMPFC) is the source of our embodied self-awareness, in which we feel sensations and emotions without cognitive labeling, and we let those feelings guide our behavioral choices.

The DMPFC and the VMPFC cannot be predominant at the same time; the neural pathways are separate, and one must switch off for the other to switch on. We are either feeling, or thinking about what we're feeling, and this distinction is reflected in the architecture of our brain.[12]

You might be thinking right about now, with all this neuroscience: How is all of this relevant to Bodymind Ballwork? Good question.

When we spend time moving slowly while feeling the pressure of the balls on the body, we are drawn into the VMPFC experience of the feeling state, the raw and direct experience of the body's sensory system. This experience has its profound benefits: we feel more deeply what the tissues of the body have to tell us, and we access our fundamental aliveness and intuition with intimacy and immediacy. Even though we might discover deep pain, we have choices. We can avoid it and work on other things for now. Or we may have an instinctive confidence that the process of working with that pain is safe at this present moment. Then after working with that pain, while reflecting on our experience and possibly describing it in words, we access the DMPFC in order to understand what that experience means and how we can make use of it. Both parts of our awareness are important. Embodied and conceptual self-awareness both help us to extract meaning from our experiences and make good choices for our own health.

Here are some words from Bessel van der Kolk that beautifully express the need for embodied self-awareness in healing from trauma:

> The only part of the brain that is capable of influencing emotional states (which are located in the limbic system) is the medial prefrontal cortex, the part that is involved with embodied introspection (i.e. attending to the inner state of the organism). The neural networks for verbal insight, understanding and planning have virtually no connecting pathways to affect the workings of the emotional brain.[13]

In order to deal with the past, traumatized people need to activate their ventromedial prefrontal cortex, which is the only part of the conscious brain that is capable of influencing emotional states. The ventromedial prefrontal cortex allows us to pay conscious attention to the internal state of the organism through a type of introspection we call embodied self-awareness. Therapy needs to help them develop a deep curiosity about their internal experience. This curiosity is essential in learning to identify their physical sensations and to translate their emotions and sensations into communicable language—communicable most of all to themselves. Once people realize that their internal sensations constantly shift and change, that they have considerable control over their physiological states, and that remembering the past does not inevitably result in overwhelming emotions, they can start to explore ways to actively influence the organization of their internal landscape. As they learn to tolerate being aware of their physical experience, they discover physical impulses and options that they had abandoned for the sake of survival during the trauma.[14]

TRUST AND AGENCY

Whether or not we have suffered trauma, we all need to feel that we can trust our body and our inner experience. Bodymind Ballwork gradually develops deeper trust in the body and trust in our capacity to access its wisdom and make changes. Even though we may be faced with situations that are out of our control (such as aging, a trauma in the past, or a current illness), we find an inner reservoir of strength and calm from working with the body in this careful, introspective way. We see that change is possible; the bodymind has plasticity, and we are always in the process of becoming.

Bessel van der Kolk writes this about agency in his book *The Body Keeps the Score:*

> Our sense of agency, how much we feel in control, is defined by our relationship with our bodies and its rhythms: our waking and sleep, and how we eat, sit, and walk define the contours of our day. In order to find our voice, we have to be in our bodies—able to breathe fully and able to access our inner sensations.[15]

Resilience is the product of agency: knowing that what you do can make a difference.[16]

Ivy Green writes in her book *Relaxation Awareness Resilience* about the deep shift in attitude toward one's body that comes from a practice like Bodymind Ballwork:

Body-focused awareness methods encourage individuals to suspend judgments and momentarily put aside the need to figure out a solution, and instead be curious about what their body's intelligence can tell them. These methods guide individuals to invite, acknowledge, befriend and trust their sensations, feelings and subtle movement shifts. Individuals learn how to listen to their body's messages with acceptance and loving attention.[17]

PART II

CHAPTER 6

Getting Started

To get started practicing the ballwork, you will obviously need a few balls. Bodymind Ballwork is done with rubber balls in several different sizes to accommodate different parts of your body and to create different amounts of pressure. Larger balls work well in areas such as knees, neck, and hips, whereas medium-sized and smaller balls are needed for the spine, shoulders, arms, abdomen, ribs, and lower legs. The smallest balls work well for the head, feet, and hands. Some balls have a different texture (soft, medium, or hard when you squeeze them); some are hollow and some are solid. Many people ask if tennis balls will work, since they are so easy to find. Although tennis balls are better than nothing, they do not adapt to the body as well as rubber balls. You can begin with a basic set of balls, which can be purchased online or in toy stores. (See the About the Author page for ordering information.)

The basic beginning set is:

- Two large hollow balls (4″-6″, about the size of a cantaloupe) for the neck, upper chest, spine, and legs

- One football-shaped ball (6″ long) for the neck, front torso, ribs, shoulders, and legs

- Two medium-sized hollow balls (3″ or 4″, about the size of a large apple or orange) for the neck, spine, arms, and legs

- Two small solid balls (2.5″-3″, about the size of a large lemon) for the spine, arms, and legs

- One small hollow ball (1.5"–2", about the size of a small lime) for the face and feet

- One very small solid ball (1"–2", about the size of a walnut) for the feet and hands

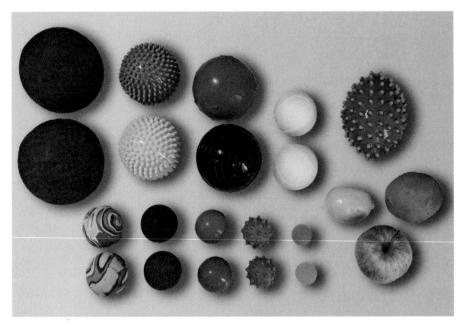

The ball collection with a lemon, an orange, and an apple at lower right for size comparison. Colors will vary.

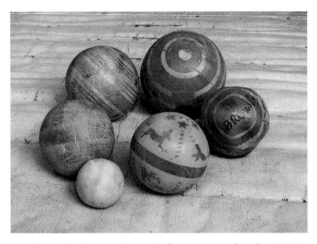

As a historical note, these balls were used in the 1960s by world-renowned choreographer Trisha Brown.

In addition to the rubber balls, you'll need a room, fairly quiet if possible, where you can lie down on the floor. A yoga mat is helpful, but not necessary. You should also have a blanket and pillow handy. If you have yoga props, include a yoga block.

It's good to have about twenty minutes or more of uninterrupted time. But the most important thing you'll need is your own permission to turn your attention inside and feel your body. With so much outward demand on our attention in the outer world of work, family, and the details of life, these conditions might be challenging. But once you develop a practice, it will become obvious how that time is well spent. Your connection with yourself will grow, making room for more self-compassion, self-understanding, and hopefully greater ease. If you have a meditation practice, you can think of ballwork as meditation with your body as the focus, and set your surroundings as you would for meditation. If you are not a meditator, you might want to choose some soothing music to help you to slow down and focus inward. You deserve this time for yourself, and it will pay off by helping you to be more present and fully available for everything else that you do.

FOCUSING INWARD

Ask yourself: What am I feeling in my body right now? Perhaps the easiest sensations might be your body position and the awareness of what is touching your skin. If you are on the floor, you can notice which parts of the body contact the floor. This is called **exteroception,** or using the five senses of touch, sight, hearing, smell, and taste to feel one's relationship to things outside the body. You might feel the texture of your clothing and the floor or carpet, or sense the temperature or light in the room. Listen to the sounds around you. Exteroception also includes feeling the boundaries of your body: Where does the outside world actually begin?

Then, taking your attention further inside, you might feel the weightedness of the body or the movement of the breath. This kind of attention is called **interoception,** or feeling sensations that come from inside the body. Further development of this kind of sensing might involve noticing your general state of energy (relaxed, agitated, or something in between), your patterns of muscular tension, your digestion, your heart rate, even your patterns of thinking. There is a vast inner world to explore.

When we move, we are using a third type of awareness called **propriocep-tion.** This is the feeling of movement, balance, and how the parts of the body arrange themselves in relation to each other. Using your proprioception, you might perceive whether your knees are bent or straight, or which way your head is turned. Proprioceptive sensors in the muscles and joints tell you when a muscle is being stretched, or when a joint is moving to its farthest range. Very slow and simple movements refine and expand your proprioception. As you enhance your proprioceptive sense, you will be able to move in a more coordinated, smooth, and efficient manner.

Every time you do ballwork, spend a few minutes first to tune into these modes of perception. Scan your outer and inner awareness as a place to start. Move a little bit to orient your perceptions to your feeling of moving. Taking time for this shift from outer to inner awareness is an important step in self-care. You are not only connecting to your physical self; you are opening to the subtle but ever-present interplay between the body, mind, and emotions. Thoughts, worries, memories, and agendas may arise. The emotions that arise might be anywhere on the spectrum from pleasant to unpleasant. This is all part of our inner experience, our inner being—no feeling is wrong.

Once you have attuned yourself to inner sensations and thoughts, you can choose a part of the body to work on with the balls. Then you can choose a technique to practice that will target that part of the body with certain balls and certain movements. In the chapters that follow, each technique is numbered and described separately with all the necessary details. There are several techniques for the shoulders, several for the spine, several for the hips, etc. I will describe the general contours of a practice session here as a preview, but please refer to subsequent chapters for specific instructions.

After placing the balls as instructed, there is a moment of settling and receiving the pressure from the balls. Take the time to feel how your body reacts, take some deep breaths, and release as much tension as you can. Let your body drape over the round shape of the balls. Then you begin to move, very slowly and gently, in a particular direction that is specific to that technique. It might be a movement of your arm or shoulder, or a movement of your ribs or hips. The slow movement combined with the pressure from the balls on the soft tissue (muscles, tendons, ligaments, and fascia) gives you the opportunity to feel that part of your body more clearly than you might have been able to feel it before. The balls dig in, and then as you move while maintaining the pressure, the balls create a shearing stretch in the layers of fascia and muscles inside. The result is happier soft tissue: less binding, better hydration and circulation, and freer movement range.

Information flows both ways: you are sensing and moving with more awareness than usual. Your movement and your perceptions inform each other. Each small adjustment of the body can be felt vividly, with the balls as a magnifying glass clarifying more details than one would in normal, everyday motion. Many students remark on this direct focusing quality of the ballwork. Some describe it as a kind of "depth probe," a nonthreatening way to locate trouble spots in the body.

The weight of your body creates pressure between you and the ball that is similar to a massage. You can adjust the pressure according to your own needs and tolerance: a smaller or softer ball gives less pressure, a larger or harder ball gives more pressure. You may feel discomfort, even pain, in certain areas at first, because of the tension your body is carrying. People also often say, "It hurts, but it's a good hurt." Tight muscles and fascia may not give way to the pressure from the ball immediately. Tension in the tissues will set off pain signals in varying degrees of intensity, which should be noticed. If the pain is agitating you, choose a softer or a smaller ball, or practice on a bed, or adapt in ways that are suggested in the instructions. As time passes, the soft tissue does soften, and you will feel satisfying pressure, but not pain. This is why I recommend having a varied selection of balls to use, so you can change the pressure as needed. You will notice that some parts of the body respond well to more pressure, and in other areas, less pressure is better. This may change from day to day as well. I encourage you to use balls that you like, because that will help you do the practice!

Most techniques in this book require about ten to twenty minutes, and a few require up to thirty minutes. Be sure to end each working session with a few minutes of rest without the balls, which allows you to notice, integrate, and assimilate the changes that have occurred. Feel your body in the areas where the balls were, but also in other areas that might have shifted or released as well. This period of integration is an essential part of the process to develop and sustain meaningful change in your experience of your body.

THE PRINCIPLES

Principle 1. Develop Awareness without Judgment

For many people, it is a new experience to observe how their body actually feels from the inside, rather than how they think it should feel, how they are afraid it might feel, or how it felt yesterday. What is going on in this very moment? Observe with as much neutrality as possible; avoid jumping into the inner conversation that judges, analyzes, or reacts to what you feel. Value curiosity over achievement. You might notice that one part of the body feels stiff, another part feels comfortable, another part feels uncomfortable in a vague or specific sort of way, and yet another part you don't feel at all. In this way, you can scan your body to see what your starting point is on any particular day.

Some of us have become accustomed to noticing only unpleasant feelings, perhaps because we take the body for granted when everything is fine. We specifically look for what hurts, or what is not working the way we want. We neglect to notice and enjoy what is feeling good. Unless something hurts, we feel "nothing."

Others might suppress the aches and pains to avoid dealing with them; areas of the body with strain or fatigue become anesthetized. The entire range of sensations is worth noticing, because we can use that feedback to learn what the body needs. As we listen more to *all* the body's messages, with some degree of objectivity, we are fine-tuning the bodymind connection and understanding ourselves more clearly. We are allowing sensations to surface that may have been censored because of pain, self-image, or assumptions or fears about the body. By being aware of the whole range of our sensations from the inside, we can make the best choices for our own health and well-being. I have found that people usually have reliable instincts. They might say to themselves: Yes, this is good for me, even if it's a bit uncomfortable at first, or No, this feels wrong and I can either stop doing it or try doing it a different way.

Principle 2. Release into Gravity

We live in the field of gravity; it is our milieu and our dance partner as we move through life. In using the balls, gravity is definitely our ally. We invite beneficial pressure into a specific part of the body by releasing our weight into the ball and draping over it. We usually will not need more pressure than that. When you first place a ball under you or against your body, take the time to release into gravity and see what happens. That simple shift can create a major change in your inner state. Take a deep breath and let yourself become heavy.

When we are stuck in a state of generalized tension and stress, the fight-or-flight response keeps us poised to meet the challenge or to run. The nervous system can become so accustomed to that state that we live that way all the time. It is remarkably calming to simply let yourself become heavy and trust that the ground will hold you. With practice, you will become more and more skilled at releasing into gravity at will.

Principle 3. Move Slowly with Minimal Effort

Moving very slowly allows us to notice and feel more subtly. It also shows us more clearly what is entailed in each movement. When we move at an ordinary speed, such as when pulling on a shirt or lifting a dish, it's unlikely that we can separate the many different sensations that accompany the action; it becomes a familiar blur with perhaps only the end result being clearly experienced. Very slow movements, however, can provide a universe of discovery. We can feel which parts of the body move easily and which parts resist movement. We may notice that we prefer certain movements to others, and the slowness helps us to interrupt the automatic patterns and find new ways to move, ones that perhaps extend our range. One way to slow yourself down is to move just a quarter of an inch, then pause to feel, then move another quarter of an inch, and another, until you've reached a natural end point to that movement.

Along with this choice about the speed of our movements, we also have a choice about the degree of effort we use. In everyday movement, we tend to use a moderate amount of effort with occasional bursts of more intensity. While walking, lifting objects, or doing tasks, we let the body naturally recruit the "right" amount of effort. Daily life usually keeps us in the middle range of effort. When we touch another person sensitively or handle a delicate object, we might scale back to a lower level of effort in our movements. When we lift something heavy, we spontaneously recruit more effort. However, sometimes that innate assessment of effort becomes disrupted, and we overdo or underdo.

For this exploration, we take the premise that using less effort will help us to understand the actual requirements for any given movement and make more efficient choices. How little or how much effort does it take to move a shoulder? Can we let go of unnecessary muscles that move only out of habit? Once the movement is done, can we release the tension that we needed to move and really feel gravity's power as it pulls our shoulder back to a rest position? You may feel the difference between moving by contracting the muscles and moving by stretching the muscles. You might also feel the difference between those times when movement is difficult and when it is easy, positions in which your body is working and those in which there is total rest. All of these discoveries will provide a closer connection between your analytic or intellectual mind and your bodymind, your conceptual self-awareness and your embodied self-awareness. With that connection, you have the skills to choose the right degree of effort for whatever you do.

As simple as they are, these slow and gentle movements may be frustrating to you, as they were to me when I began to do this work. Many of us are accustomed to moving quickly and without very much thought, or moving to create a certain visual or functional effect. The internal focus of exploring movement for its own sake may be a new experience, one that is fascinating and liberating.

Principle 4. Explore Your Range

Often in daily life, our movements are restricted to habitual patterns that we repeat over and over because they are functional. If you think about your daily life, you can easily think of positions and movements that are so familiar and frequent that you don't notice how they feel.

When practicing the ballwork, you can have the intention to feel those ordinary movements more fully. For instance, when working with your shoulder, invite yourself to investigate all the different directions the shoulder can move. What does it feel like in the joint and the surrounding muscles when you raise your arm up overhead? When you initiate the movement from your shoulder blade, instead of from the arm or hand? When you move your arm across the body as far as possible? When you reach back? When you turn the arm in different directions?

Exploring in this way can reawaken pathways of connection in your bodymind and give you more range of movement than you thought you had. You'll be filling in your **body schema**—the detailed but also unifying knowledge of the boundaries of the body, the movements you can do with each part, and how the parts relate to each other. You'll see how each part moving affects every other part in some way. When you move your arm, your neck and torso will probably register that movement in some way. Every part is connected, and yet every part can move on its own. This experiential realization is very empowering, especially after an injury, when we might tend to avoid moving out of fear.

By narrowing the field of attention and focusing on a specific joint or area of the body, you can sense more details about how you move, and you can begin to recognize interrelationships. One student who had a shoulder injury told me, "When I began, I rarely moved my shoulders, especially my left shoulder, alone. My neck, even my back, wanted to get in on the act." Her injury exacerbated a habitual movement pattern established at least in part by her work at her computer.

Moving one part of the body by itself is a skill that underlies a good, self-supporting alignment—that is, a balanced arrangement of each of the parts of the body in relation to the others. With sound alignment, you will have maximum strength and flexibility and be able to move easily, at will, with small adjustments exactly where and when they are needed to perform a particular gesture or task. This is the secret of good posture that allows safe, energy-efficient movement.

THE BREATH IS THE LINK

The breath is a natural—and useful—bridge between the mind and the body. Remember the second kosha, pranamaya kosha, the body of breath? Our breath continues without our conscious direction every moment of our lives, and yet we can choose to notice it and work with it. The intention to become more familiar and fluent with our own breath is an immensely powerful means of self-regulation. We can recharge when we are tired, or de-stress when that is what we need.

Sue, who is a pianist, noticed how much her sense of musical rhythm was influenced by her breathing patterns; when she was anxious, or concentrating on difficult passages, her breathing would be unsteady and her rhythm askew. With greater awareness of her breath, she was able to be steadier in her playing.

It is natural for such changes in the breathing to happen. In some cases, changes in breathing can be beneficial—such as when running for a bus or during childbirth. But sometimes the disturbance or change in breathing remains after its initial cause has passed. You can probably think of times when your breath was strained by an exertion, or constricted by anger or fear. Did it return to an easeful state after the stress had passed? Or was there a residue that remained?

While working with the balls, be aware of your normal breath, and allow it to adapt and shift as you explore. Notice the many possible qualities of breath. You might feel your breath as pleasant, nourishing, uneven, steady, fluid, restricted, or expansive. These are just some examples; observe what you feel, moment by moment. When you feel discomfort from the pressure of the balls, take a deep breath to aid the process of release and change. When the ball feels good, enjoy it and take a deep breath to savor that enjoyment! The spontaneous deeper breath that often happens as a result of using the balls is delicious, and marks an authentic connection to your true self.

The effects of working with the breath can be specific or general, dramatic or subtle. Your spine may lengthen, your shoulders and chest may relax, your voice may deepen, your mind may become clearer. Your whole body may feel lighter or heavier. Whatever the response, easier breathing always brings easier movement and a greater feeling of well-being, because the breath is quite literally a foundation of being alive.

ABOVE ALL, TRUST YOURSELF

Trust yourself to choose the right balls, the right parts of the body to work on, and the right duration of your practice. Trust yourself to gradually understand and integrate the process and the results. Doing the practice regularly will teach you how to deepen, how to expand, how to use it most fully for your own benefit. Trust your bodymind to reveal to you what you need to know for healing, for inner and outer realignment, for easeful movement and self-fulfillment.

The next chapters provide detailed instructions for ballwork techniques, addressing virtually every part of the body. Now that you've prepared yourself with knowledge of the basic principles of Bodymind Ballwork, you're ready to get started!

CHAPTER 7

The Best Basic Everyday Practices

Imagine your spine as supple and strong, enabling you to stand tall and to move through your day with ease. Though "good" posture may have previously been arduous or unattainable, you begin to feel your posture improving without effort as your muscles release unnecessary tension. Your hips move fluidly, and your feet are solidly on the ground. Imagine your breath as expansive and nourishing, your ribs moving easily as your lungs fill and empty. With a steady and satisfying breath, your mind stays calm and alert, and you can focus on whatever you need to attend to, with full attention and clarity.

Does that scenario seem possible to you? It might seem like a distant goal if you are accustomed to chronic neck, shoulder, or lower back pain, as so many people are. You will find, though, that you can reduce or even eliminate that pain with the help of the balls. If you have certain spots in your back that are always nagging at your awareness with a "hot spot" or a dull ache, you have the chance to change that pattern, target those spots, and provide yourself with relief. Sore feet? Relief could be just ten minutes away.

Daily practice of the six basic techniques included in this chapter will dramatically change your experience of your body. As your body carries less tension on a daily basis, you move more easily, your energy is sustainable, and you sleep more soundly.

You can practice these techniques in any order, and you can choose one or two to get started. Once you have tried them all, you can make your own sequences that address what you most need.

1. THE NECK

When you are first learning the ballwork, the neck is an excellent place to begin. Tension in the neck can be the beginning of many common discomforts—muscle and joint stiffness, eyestrain, mental fatigue, and headaches. Ballwork on the neck can help to ease tension in the jaw and face, and even have benefits down into the arms and hands. For those who spend a lot of time in front of a computer screen, it is essential.

Ball: One hollow ball, 4″ or 5″ or the football-shaped ball

Body position: Lying on your back, with your legs stretched out, or knees bent

Starting position of the ball: At the top of your neck, just below the edge of your skull. Your forehead will be higher than your chin.

Action: Allow the weight of your head to fully rest on the ball. Then very slowly turn your head to one side, feeling each small area that you pass over. Take your time! Linger in any spot that feels tight, possibly adding a nodding motion to explore more range. As you get farther to the side, you can move the ball over a bit with your hand, to keep your head securely on top of the ball. Once your head is turned as far as is comfortable, take a breath or two, and then slowly bring your head back to center. Let your head rest here for a few moments and then do the same slow exploration on the other side. Take a few breaths, relaxing in the center, before moving on. At any time, you may improvise a direction of movement that feels possible to explore. For instance, while your head is centered, you could try a nodding motion to feel the spine moving against the pressure of the ball.

Progression: Move the ball down an inch or so, under the middle of your neck. Your chin and forehead will be level here. Then move your head very slowly to one side and then back to center. Once back to center, take a few breaths and then repeat to the other side. After you bring your head back to center again, relax for a moment. Again, try the nodding motion while your head is centered.

At the third spot, your chin will be higher than your forehead, and your head will tilt back behind the ball. You're working on the lower part of your neck (C4–C6), where the neck may be more stiff than it was farther up toward your head. Adjust with a smaller ball if necessary. Repeat the same process, taking your time.

The fourth spot on the neck is on C7, the lowest cervical vertebra at the base of the neck. This bone is more prominent than the ones above, so you may need a softer or a slightly smaller ball. Now your movement will be a shift or a lean from side to side, because there is limited rotation at this level of your spine. Working on this spot helps to integrate the neck into the upper back.

Duration: 10–15 minutes

Contraindications: Recent cervical disk herniation, cervical instability, extreme dizziness

Notes: It's fine to work on only the first two spots if your neck is short or the lower spots are not comfortable. Notice possible effects in your sinuses, jaw, eyes, forehead, or shoulders. Working on your neck has many possible benefits—sometimes unexpected—and it is a fundamental practice for calming and centering the mind.

Anatomy: Cervical vertebral segments, suboccipital muscles, cervical transversospinalis muscles, cervical portions of the erector spinae, splenius capitis, upper trapezius

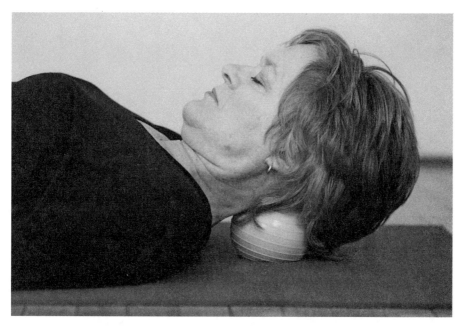

The Neck, Ball Position 1

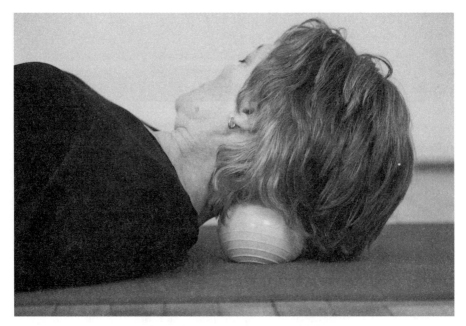

The Neck, Ball Position 1, Turning

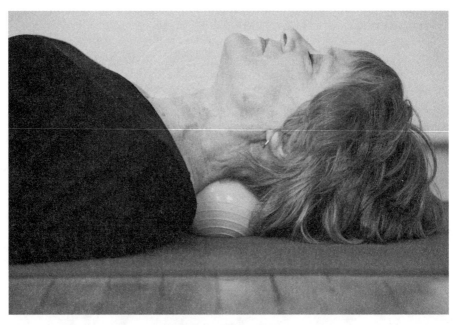

The Neck, Ball Position 2

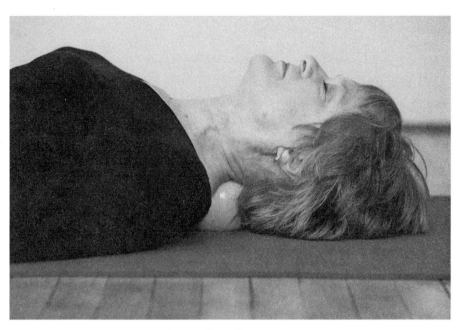

The Neck, Ball Position 3

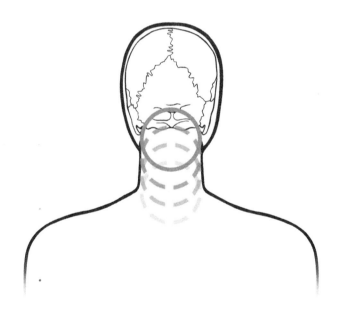

Ball Placement for the Neck

2. THE TRAPEZIUS

Tension around the tops of the shoulders plagues just about everyone I know. Stress builds here in the form of muscle tension, whether it's from carrying bags or children, worrying, hurrying, having less than ideal posture, or getting inadequate sleep—just to name a few possible causes. Softening the trapezius muscle does a huge service to your state of mind and increases comfort throughout your body. You'll feel different after just one session, and even better if you practice this every day.

Balls: Two solid or hollow balls, 2.5″. You might also use a folded blanket, bolster, or yoga block during this technique (see Variation).

Body position: Lying on your back with your legs straight or bent

Starting position of the balls: One on each side, at the very top of your upper back, in the area of soft tissue of the upper trapezius muscle, between your shoulders and your neck

Action: Movement 1: Position your arms with the elbows pointing upward, hands resting on your forehead or behind your head. Move your elbows slowly up toward the ceiling with your hands still touching your forehead. This movement comes from your shoulder blades moving around from the back to the sides of your ribs (protraction). Each time you release your arms down, allow the muscles to soften around the balls.

Movement 2: First, place a folded blanket behind you in case you need support for your arms. Extend your arms overhead onto the blanket. Shift your shoulders and upper back slowly to one side, then back to center, then slowly to the other side. Repeat as many times as you wish.

Move slowly and linger in any spot that feels particularly tight. Take some deep breaths and picture the muscles melting around the ball.

An alternate arm position is to cross your arms over your chest, creating more pressure.

Progression: Move the balls slightly wider apart or closer together and repeat the actions. Then move the balls an inch or two down your back, between the shoulder blades, and repeat all the actions. Continue moving the balls down one spot at a time, until you reach the bottom corner of the shoulder blades. Usually you will find four spots. Try each of the arm positions to see which one works well for you.

Duration: 15-20 minutes

Contraindications: Try this for a short time as a test if you have a recent neck or shoulder injury, shoulder subluxation, nerve entrapment, repetitive strain injury (RSI), cervical disk herniation, or labral tear. Stop if your pain increases from the pressure of the ball. This technique will help to relieve secondary spasms that follow shoulder and neck injuries, so it is worth testing it.

Variation: For more pressure at the upper trapezius, repeat movement 2 with your knees bent and your hips raised on a folded blanket, bolster, or yoga block. This lift of your hips will change the angle of pressure and reach some additional trigger points in the upper trapezius muscle.

Anatomy: Trapezius, semispinalis capitis, splenius capitis and cervicis, levator scapulae, rhomboids, intercostals

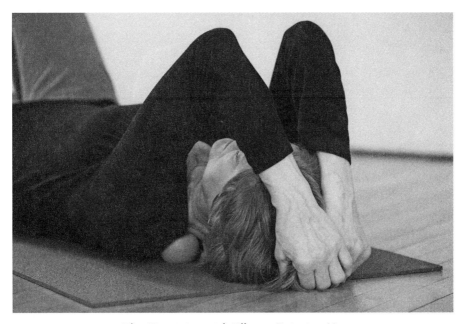

The Trapezius with Elbows Pointing Up

Many students say that these two techniques—The Neck and The Trapezius—are lifesavers. Aliza, the executive director of a nonprofit corporation, had done many years of regular yoga practice when she developed severe neck pain and numbness in her arms, making her wary of continuing her yoga. Massage and acupuncture helped, but eventually a diagnosis of herniated disks in her cervical spine took her to spinal surgeons who wanted to schedule her for immediate spinal fusion in her neck. She decided to try adding ballwork to her regular practice. "The first private class was a revelation! The ballwork made me feel immediate relief much as the massage and acupuncture had, but I could do it at home and with greater frequency. And I could practice yoga again. I take a class that combines ballwork and yoga poses weekly and try to take out the balls at home several times a week—especially when I feel stiff. I have now been practicing yoga combined with ballwork for about four years. It has helped to improve my posture and has given me almost full relief from pain. More than anything, it is empowering. If my neck tenses, I don't go into a tailspin of 'what ifs.' I know it is time to grab my balls and blocks, lie down on the floor, and relieve the pain."

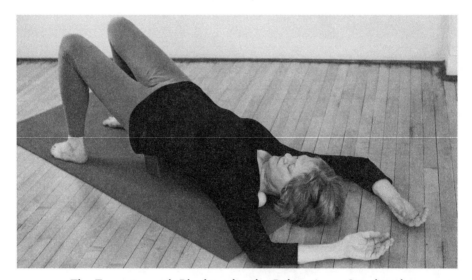

The Trapezius with Block under the Pelvis, Arms Overhead

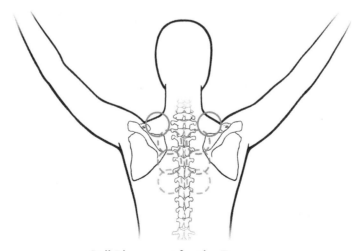

Ball Placement for the Trapezius

3. THE SPINE WITH TWO BALLS

With this technique, you can reach the large muscles of the middle and lower back that are often the source of fatigue and pain. Use it in combination with The Trapezius technique (above) and The Back of the Pelvis technique (below) if you want to work from the shoulders down through the pelvis. As a daily practice, this one will help to prevent incipient musculoskeletal back problems from developing, and your breathing will improve.

Balls: Two balls, either 2.5″ solid balls or 3″–4″ hollow balls (smooth or spiky). Solid balls will penetrate more, so choose those if you like deep pressure. Hollow balls will still loosen your muscles, but with less intense pressure.

Body position: Lying on your back, with your knees bent or straight, whichever is more comfortable for you

Starting position of the balls: Just below your shoulder blades, one on each side of the spine

Action: Settle yourself on the balls, taking several deep breaths. Then begin to move your spine and ribs very slowly to one side. Take your time and feel each small gradation of movement. Then return to center and pause to breathe. Slowly move to the other side, moving only that part of your spine and ribs. Do as many repetitions from side to side as you wish. Try to move just the part of the spine where the balls are touching, and avoid pushing with your legs.

Progression: Move the balls down an inch or two on your back, either with your hands or by letting them roll as you shift your body in the direction of your head. Repeat the movements at this new spot. Continue down your entire spine, one spot at a time, until you feel the top of your pelvis in contact with the balls.

Be attentive to your breath, especially when working in the midback, near the diaphragm.

Duration: 15–20 minutes

Contraindications: Recent disk herniation, or spinal fracture. For those with spinal stenosis and scoliosis: My experience is that this technique is very beneficial, but I encourage you to use your own best judgment. Try it for a few sessions and see if you feel more ease in your posture and movement.

Notes: You may need one type of ball on the upper part of the spine and a different type lower down, due to the tension patterns in your back. Feel free to change the balls if necessary.

Anatomy: Thoracic and lumbar vertebral segments, the erector spinae and quadratus lumborum muscles, the lumbosacral fascia, and indirectly the diaphragm muscle and the iliopsoas muscle

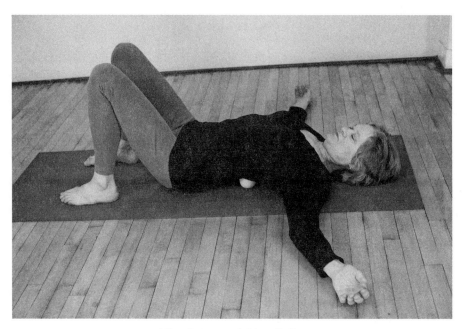

The Spine with Two Balls

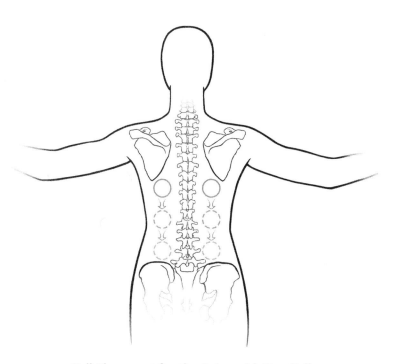

Ball Placement for the Spine with Two Balls

4. THE BACK OF THE PELVIS

We sit on our hips and buttocks every day, yet we hardly feel the layers of muscles that are there. This technique will show you the tight spots and let you work on them slowly and gradually so that your pelvic muscles have a more even tone. People report relief from sciatic pain, piriformis syndrome, sacroiliac pain, general low backache, and PMS when these muscles release in response to the balls. There's also a grounding and settling effect on the entire nervous system. From the yogic point of view, this technique increases apana vayu, the downward flowing prana that brings steadiness and calm.

Balls: Two balls, either hollow or solid, 2.5″–4″ in diameter

Body position: Lying on your back, knees bent

Starting position of the balls: Under the center of your buttocks, one ball on each side

Action: Begin by taking time to release your weight into the balls and compare the sensations on each side. Then start to move very slowly in any direction. Explore a side-to-side direction, an up-and-down direction, diagonals, and any other variation that you can do. Move the pelvis by itself rather than pushing with your legs. Work on one small area at a time, moving in different directions to change the angle of pressure from the balls.

Progression: Work the middle spot first, to get used to the feeling of the balls in this area. Then work systematically through the entire back of your pelvis, one spot at a time in this way: Place the balls high on the buttocks, near your waist. Find several spots here, at first close to the center, then wider apart, then even wider apart.

Move the balls lower, toward the middle of your buttocks, and in close to the midline. Progress to two or three spots farther to the sides.

Then work on the lowest row of spots, from your tailbone in the center, and progressing to the sides of the lower buttocks.

When you have explored the entire area, you can go back to a spot that felt good as an ending.

Variations:

1. For deeper pressure, bring one knee toward your chest and then to the side.

2. "Windshield wiper": Widen your feet, then tilt one bent knee down and across toward your opposite foot, turning the thigh inward. This will bring more pressure to the opposite side from the knee that comes down.

3. Ankle to knee: Place one ankle over the opposite knee to create more pressure on the piriformis muscle.

4. Sit almost upright with your knees bent, leaning back a bit onto your hands. Work the balls into the lower buttocks, all around the sitting bones. Raising the upper body in this way will give you more pressure than when you are lying down.

With all these variations, place the legs as indicated and then move your pelvis slowly to one side and then the other.

Duration: 15-20 minutes

Contraindications: Extreme nerve pain, either in the buttocks or down the legs

Anatomy: Sacrum, sacroiliac joint and its ligaments, lumbosacral fascia, gluteus maximus, gluteus medius, gluteus minimus, piriformis, gemellus inferior and superior, obturator internus, sacrotuberous ligament

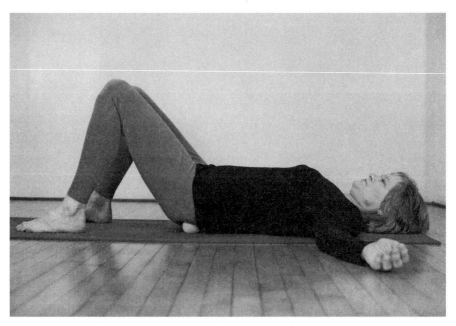

The Back of the Pelvis

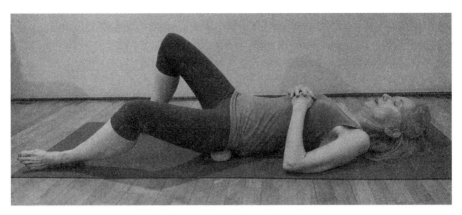

The Back of the Pelvis Variation 1

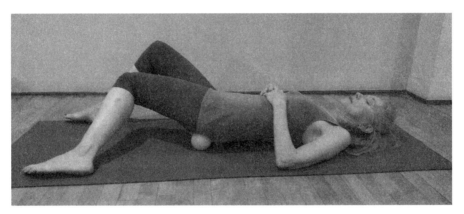

The Back of the Pelvis Variation 2

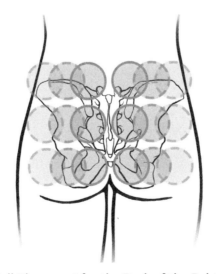

Ball Placement for the Back of the Pelvis

5. THE FRONT OF THE HIPS

Like the previous technique, this one is also very calming and grounding, and it increases apana vayu, the downward flowing prana in the body. This part of the body, the juncture of the upper body and the legs, is a common repository of physical and mental stress. Long car or plane trips, intense yoga practices, running, and general anxiety all tend to cause tightening here. As the hip flexor muscles release, the thighs shift back, the diaphragm releases, and the breath deepens. Try this one at the beginning, middle, or end of your day, and you'll be glad you did. It's gentle and yet it works very deeply.

Balls: Two 4" or 5" hollow balls

Body position: Lying face down with optional padding for your head and shoulders. Your head can face straight down resting on your hands, or you can turn it to the side.

Starting position of the balls: Under the front hip sockets, more to the sides than at the center. If you feel any numbness or a strong pulse, move the balls wider apart.

Action: Settle your weight into the balls and breathe, letting your pelvis drape over the balls. Your lower back will arch slightly from this support. If you feel your pulse strongly, move the balls wider apart to avoid pressing onto large blood vessels.

When you are ready, move slowly to one side, back to center, then to the other side, taking your time. Pause wherever it feels interesting to explore further.

Variations:

1. Pelvic tilt, moving your tailbone up and then down.

2. Roll the legs inward and then outward, by turning heels out and then in.

3. Lengthen one leg out away from your pelvis, while shortening the other one.

Progression: Move the balls up or down an inch or two to a different spot and repeat these movements.

Duration: 10-15 minutes

Contraindications: Recent hip or abdominal surgery, labral tear, late pregnancy, ischial bursitis

Notes: Take time to breathe during this one; it encourages a release of the diaphragm and is very calming to the breath and the mind. Avoid neck strain by turning your head frequently.

If your pelvis is torqued, you can help to adjust it by placing the balls asymmetrically on your front hips. Place the ball higher on the side that tends to tilt anteriorly (arching the lumbar spine), and the ball lower on the side that tends to tilt posteriorly (tucking under).

Anatomy: Inguinal ligament, iliopsoas, rectus femoris, sartorius

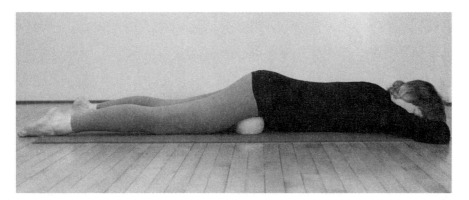

The Front of the Hips

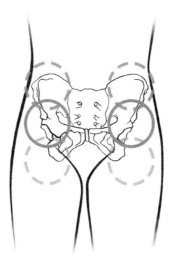

Ball Placement for the Front of the Hips

6. THE SOLES OF THE FEET

We take our feet for granted, and sometimes stuff them into shoes that look great but feel uncomfortable or don't support the feet well at all. We all have virtually the same anatomy in the bones and muscles, yet there is infinite variety in how all these parts function. Our feet develop in response to how they are used, or misused, or underused. I see many people who say they have flat feet, and often tell me stories about other family members whose feet are the same. Yet when I look at their feet while standing and also without bearing weight, very often their arches are not flat, but actually weak and distorted by poor alignment. The arches collapse down and the weight is randomly distributed, often with associated tensions in the lower legs.

Because our feet carry the whole weight of the body, they need to be supple, strong, and intelligent—able to appropriately respond to the ever-changing demands of daily life. The first step in reeducating the feet is to really feel them, and feel the floor under you more fully. See where the sore spots are, and investigate the effects that tightness may have on your posture. How does your walk feel different after doing a few minutes of work on your feet? People often say they feel lighter, more connected to the earth, calmer, and more aware of the way they carry weight on the feet. Your balance improves as your feet become more intelligent and aware. Pain from plantar fasciitis can be relieved. Practicing this technique for the soles of the feet is a starting point on the journey to feel, strengthen, and appreciate your feet more.

Ball: One small solid or hollow ball, 1″–2″

Body position: Standing, with support of a wall or chair nearby if necessary for balance support. Alternatively, you can do this technique while sitting.

Starting position of the ball: Under the front and center of the foot, near the base of the toes. Keep your heel on the floor.

Action: Allow your foot to release and drape over the ball. Put as much pressure into the ball as you wish, but only with your body weight. Then begin to tilt your foot slowly to vary the angle of pressure. Tip in all directions, working on this one spot very thoroughly. You can also roll side to side a small amount. Always keep one part of your foot on the floor to avoid moving too fast.

Progression: Follow this pathway to reach all parts of the foot, working each spot carefully: From the starting point, progress one spot at a time toward your heel. There will be about five or six spots to work on in that centerline of your foot. Then work onto the heel, with the ball of your foot stabilized on the floor. Make your way across your heel and then work your way up to the toes, one spot at a time, along the outer edge of your foot. Then with your heel back on the floor, make your way across the toes, and down the inner edge of your foot. Finish with your favorite spot, and then repeat the sequence on your other foot.

Duration: 10 minutes per foot

Contraindications: Recent fracture

Notes: When finished with your first foot, pause to stand and walk, noticing the difference between your two feet. Also notice the effects farther up your body, into your legs and the whole side of your body. Notice how increased sensitivity in your feet allows you to carefully adjust your stance and your gait.

Anatomy: All the bones, muscles, and fascia of the feet, especially the plantar fascia, flexor digitorum brevis, abductor digiti minimi, abductor hallucis, and quadratus plantae

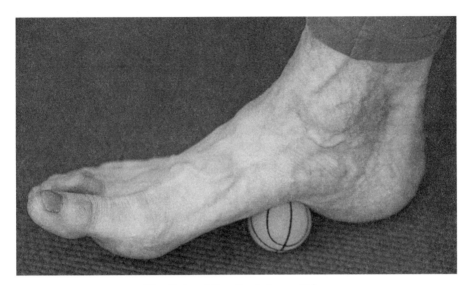

The Sole of the Foot, Inner Edge

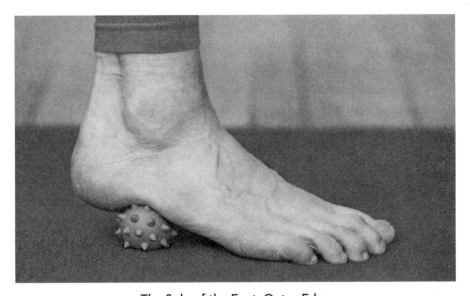

The Sole of the Foot, Outer Edge

These four techniques—The Spine with Two Balls, The Back of the Pelvis, The Front of the Hips, and The Soles of the Feet—all give a sense of groundedness. The release of outer tension in these keys areas brings our attention inward to a steady center, and a literal connection to the steadiness of the earth. Alice describes her experience: "In the course of daily life, my back tends to tighten up and gradually I have a vicious cycle of discomfort—and sometimes pain—mixed with a feeling of anxiety, distraction, and fatigue. When I work with the balls on my back, hips, and feet, I feel a powerful connection to the ground under me. It's very calming and centering. Sometimes I do it at the beginning of the day to wake up my body awareness, sometimes in the middle as a welcome break, and sometimes at the end of the day to release the residue of any stresses that day. It's amazing how much difference twenty minutes on the balls can make to my state of mind and my energy."

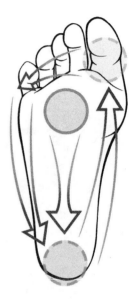

**Ball Placement for the
Sole of the Foot**

CHAPTER 8

The Spine

When your back is aching, it's hard to concentrate or to bring full enthusiasm and energy to whatever your day entails. A few minutes spent with the balls under your back can make the difference between a day that you endure and a day that you enjoy. The techniques described here supplement the basic technique presented in chapter 7, with two balls on the sides of the spine. Use these to treat spot areas of tension and pain, or to integrate your whole spine so that it moves fluidly. It will be sure to change your state of mind and your posture for the better! One student reported, "My spine feels more enlivened than it has ever felt in my entire life!" with a big smile on her face.

1. THE SPINE WITH THREE BALLS

This technique is gentle, with the pressure spread among three balls of equal size. It's a good one to do for a quick recharge when you're under stress, or you've been sitting for a long time.

Balls: Three hollow 3″ or 4″ balls, either soft or firm according to your preference

Body position: Lying on your back with your legs stretched out or knees bent, arms comfortably by your side. Have a folded towel or small cushion handy in case you need it under your head in the beginning.

Starting position of the balls: Under your upper ribs, arranged in a triangle with the single ball on your spine, and the other two below that one, on each side of the spine. Leave about an inch between balls to allow them to move. Place the folded towel under your head and neck if you need support there.

Action: Take a few minutes to relax onto the balls and settle your energy and your breath. Observe any sensations in your back, ribs, and chest. Then begin to move your spine and ribs very slowly to one side. Take time to feel each small gradation of movement. Then return to center and pause to breathe. Slowly move to the other side, moving only that part of your spine and ribs that touch the balls. Do as many repetitions from side to side as you wish.

Progression: Move the balls down an inch or two on your back, either with your hands or by letting them roll as you shift your body in the direction of your head. Repeat the movements at this new spot. Continue down your entire spine, one spot at a time, until you feel the top of your pelvis in contact with the balls. At any point you can remove the two balls that are side by side, or the single ball above them, in order to feel more pressure from the balls.

Be attentive to your breath, especially when working in the midback, near the diaphragm. Avoid overusing your abdominal muscles, although they will be involved.

Duration: 10-15 minutes

Contraindications: Recent disk herniation or spinal surgery. For scoliosis and spinal stenosis, use your own discretion.

Notes: Remind yourself to take deep breaths often. Because this technique releases tension in the ribs, your breath will change.

Anatomy: Intercostals, deep intervertebral muscles, diaphragm, erector spinae, quadratus lumborum

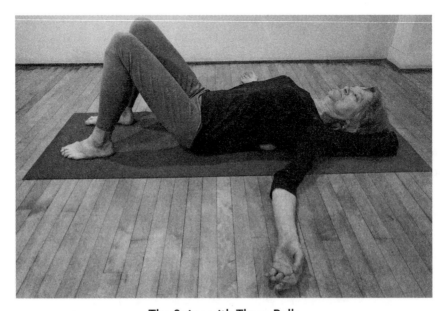

The Spine with Three Balls

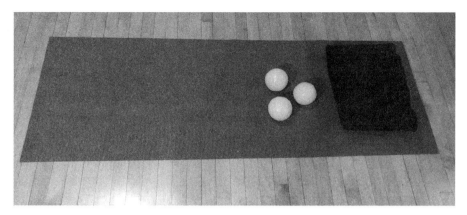

Ball Position for the Spine with Three Balls

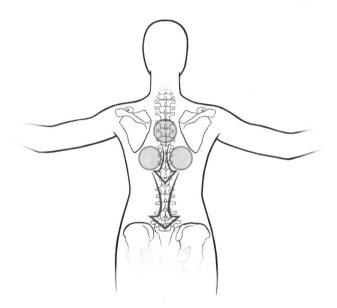

Ball Placement for the Spine with Three Balls

2. THE SPINE WITH TWO BALLS VERTICALLY

In this technique, both balls are directly on the spine. It's a good one for anyone with kyphosis (rounding of the spine) as it encourages spinal extension but in a gentle way because the pressure is spread between two balls. Use it to open up particular areas of your back that are stuck in a forward bend, as in a slouch or dowager's hump. In this case, be sure to support your head with a folded towel or blanket as needed.

Balls: Two hollow 4″ balls of equal size and texture. If you are quite stiff, start with soft balls and progress to firmer ones when you're ready.

Body position: Lying on your back. Knees can be bent or straight, arms to the sides or overhead. You may want to support your head with a folded towel or blanket. If the pressure on your spine is too intense, choose softer or smaller balls.

Starting position of the balls: Under the upper back, between the shoulder blades, in a vertical line on the spine

Action: Begin by breathing and releasing your body weight into the floor. See if you can avoid bracing yourself against the pressure from the balls; let your spine arch. Once you have settled, begin to move your spine very slowly to one side, breathing continuously. Feel the change in pressure and contact points as you move. Then move back to center and pause to take another breath. Move to the other side, feeling all sensations that accompany the movement. Then continue to move from side to side several more times.

Progression: Move the balls down an inch or two on your back, either with your hands or by letting them roll as you shift your body in the direction of your head. Repeat the movements at this new spot. Continue down your entire spine, working with one area at a time.

Duration: 10-15 minutes

Contraindications: Recent disk herniation or spinal surgery. For scoliosis and spinal stenosis, try this technique for a session or two, and then evaluate the result.

Notes: Choose balls that give you enough pressure to encourage release but that are not hard enough to cause pain.

Anatomy: Intervertebral segments, including disks, ligaments, fascia, muscles, and tendons, especially interspinales

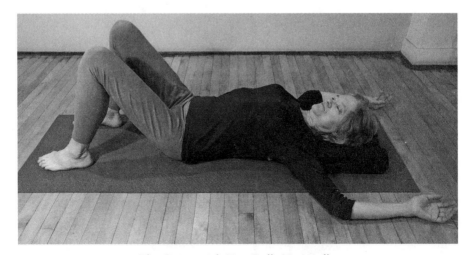

The Spine with Two Balls Vertically

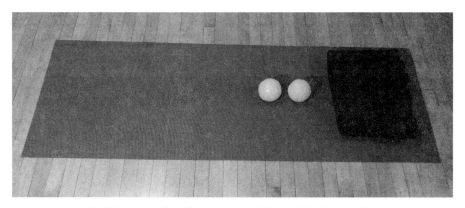

Ball Position for the Spine with Two Balls Vertically

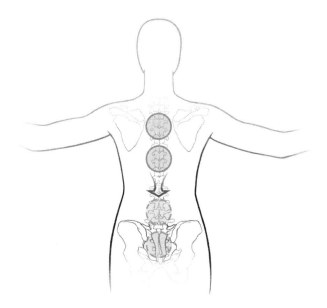

Ball Placement for the Spine with Two Balls Vertically

3. THE SPINE WITH ONE BALL

Now you'll be using just one ball directly on the spine, so choose carefully according to your preference for pressure. I use this technique as a follow-up to the other spine techniques, to consolidate gains in mobility and segmental freedom.

Ball: One hollow ball, 4″, 5″, or 6″, or the football-shaped ball

Body position: On your back, with knees bent or straight, arms anywhere they're comfortable, support under your head if needed

Starting position of the ball: Under the upper thoracic spine

Action: Give yourself time to settle, adjusting the placement of the ball as needed and possibly putting support under your head for the first few spots. Then move that part of your spine very slowly to one side, shifting your torso laterally. Linger on that side for a moment, and then slowly return to center. Then move slowly to the other side in the same way. Repeat this sequence as many times as you wish.

Progression: Roll your body over the ball to progress to the next spot, about 2″ farther down your spine. Stay there and move from side to side several times, slowly and smoothly. If the movement becomes jerky, pause and slow down, thinking of the movement as easeful exploration rather than as a task to be completed. Continue down your spine, ending with the ball under your sacrum.

Duration: 15-20 minutes

Contraindications: Recent disk herniation or spinal surgery. For scoliosis and spinal stenosis, try this technique for a session or two, and then evaluate the result.

Notes: Choose balls that give you enough pressure to encourage release but that are not hard enough to cause pain.

Anatomy: Intervertebral segments, including disks, ligaments, fascia, muscles, and tendons, especially interspinales

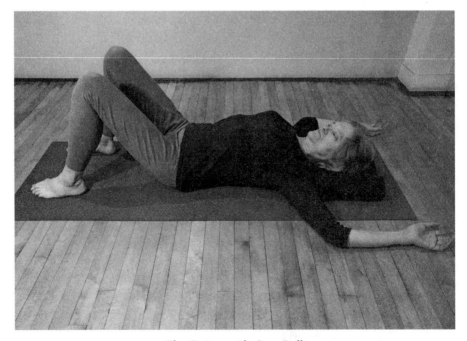

The Spine with One Ball

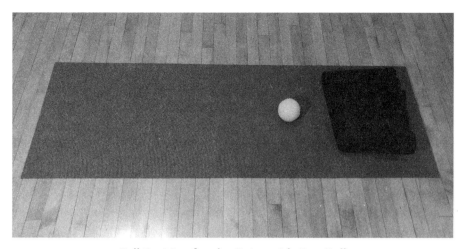

Ball Position for the Spine with One Ball

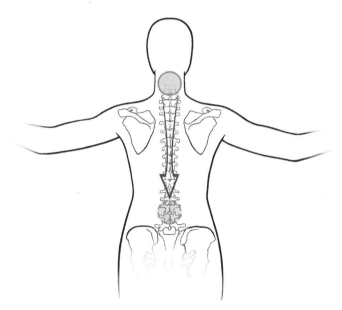

Ball Placement for the Spine with One Ball

4. THE SPINE WITH TWO LARGE BALLS, LEGS SUPPORTED (AS IN SETU BANDHASANA, BRIDGE POSE, WITH LEGS UP)

Again, the balls are directly on the spine, but this time we use the large 5″ balls, which give the feeling of floating. If you want a few minutes of bliss before meditation or sleep, or to recharge after exertion, this is a good one.

Balls: Two large 5″ hollow balls

Body position: Lying on your back, near a bed, chair, or couch that can support your legs

Starting position of the balls: One under your sacrum, the other under your lower thoracic spine

Action: Once you are settled, make very small and slow movements from side to side.

Progression: The balls can stay in the starting position, or you can make small adjustments to reach nearby spots.

Duration: 10 minutes

Contraindications: Recent spinal or abdominal surgery, vertigo, high blood pressure

Notes: Warning: You may fall asleep!

Anatomy: Sacrum, lumbar and thoracic spinal segments, small intervertebral muscles, lumbar fascia

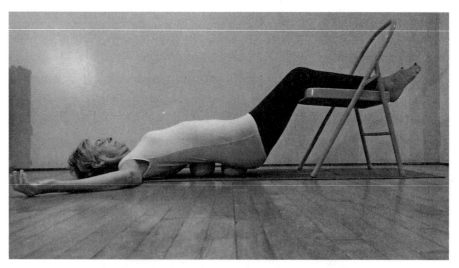

The Spine with Two Large Balls, Legs Supported

These techniques for the spine are especially good for improving posture. It's common—especially with long hours in front of a computer—for the upper back to become rounded in kyphosis ("hunchback"). Not only can this cause muscular pain and difficulties with breathing, but it is a significant risk factor for osteoporotic fractures. My students have reported that their posture improved by working directly on the spine, and they've been better able to strengthen the back with the new awareness that this work brings. Susan, a retired teacher, says this: "I had tremendous tension in my upper back that was causing terrible pain in my neck and shoulders. Doctors wanted to give me a nerve block, but I wanted to try other things first. The ballwork has increased my awareness—I can actually feel the parts of my spine so much more clearly—and my range of motion is so much better. I use the balls regularly to keep the tension from building up again. My upper back and ribs were completely stiff before, and now I can move them and feel them. It is a huge change and very empowering."

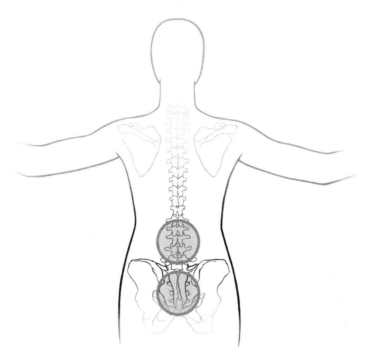

Ball Placement for the Spine with Two Large Balls, Legs Supported

CHAPTER 9

The Neck, Head, and Face

The techniques in this chapter supplement two of the techniques for the neck and shoulders that are outlined in chapter 7: The Neck and The Trapezius techniques. If you have chronic neck pain, frequent headaches, jaw tension, or eye fatigue, I recommend that you try these techniques over a period of a week or two, and see if you find relief.

1. THE SIDE OF THE NECK

We often don't notice tightness in the side of the neck, but these muscles are constantly at work as we turn our head or support it when it is off center. Your head may be off center most of the time if you have scoliosis, or if your daily activities or exercise routines require head and neck movements. If you bicycle, practice yoga, play a sport like soccer, racquetball, or tennis, or sit at a computer for long hours, your neck is working hard, even though your attention might go to your legs or shoulders.

It's worth doing some focused self-observation to begin. Take a moment to look in the mirror (without judgment!) and observe a few things. Is your head centered over your torso? You can see how your nose lines up over your sternum.

Does your head tend to turn to one side? This could be from habit, from a spinal torsion, or from an adjustment to your eyesight; a person with better vision in one eye may turn their head to favor that side.

Is there a difference in contour between the left and right sides of your neck? When the head is carried off center, the muscles will develop asymmetrically.

The nerves of your arms exit from the spinal cord in the lower neck (C5, C6, C7), often through the scalene muscles in a structure called the brachial plexus, which this technique focuses on. Many of my students with repetitive strain injury have found relief with this technique. When the scalene muscles release, there is less chance of pressure on the brachial plexus, the nerves that go down your arms.

Ball: One 4″ or 5″ ball, or the football-shaped ball

Body position: Lying on your side, with a pad under your ribs and a small pad under your head. Your shoulder has space between the two pads. You might want a bolster or pillow to support your top leg. The pad under your ribs spans the distance between your armpit and your pelvic bones. The pad under your head is the right size (when combined with the ball) to support your head and neck in a straight line with your spine and pelvis.

Starting position of the ball: Under the side of the neck

Action: Take time to arrange yourself comfortably on your side, with enough padding to have your head, chest, and pelvis in a neutral alignment. Settle yourself with a few deep breaths, and see if the ball you have chosen is appropriate for you (not too hard or too soft, too big or too small).

When you are ready, begin to turn your head very slowly toward the floor, bringing the contact with the ball more to the front of your neck. Avoid pressing on your windpipe. Then turn your head slowly back to center and pause. Then slowly turn your head toward the ceiling. At any point, you can do a nodding motion or move your head diagonally, varying the angle of pressure on the specific spot you are working with. Movements are very small and slow, to allow for more complete sensing and for release. Notice sensations in other parts of your neck, as well as in your face, jaw, and shoulders.

Progression: You may be able to move the ball a bit higher or a bit lower on your neck, depending on the length of your neck and the size of the ball. If so, try these additional placements of the ball in the same way, turning your head slowly down toward the floor and up toward the ceiling.

Duration: 5-10 minutes per side

Contraindications: Cervical subluxation

Notes: Notice your response to the pressure of the ball as you work. If you are resisting the release of your head and neck into gravity, try working with a smaller or softer ball.

Anatomy: Scalenes (anterior, middle, and posterior), upper trapezius, sternocleidomastoid

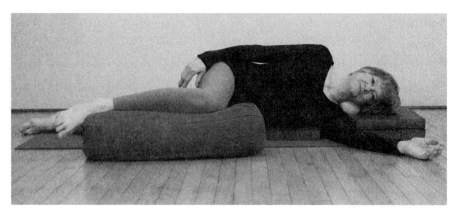

The Side of the Neck

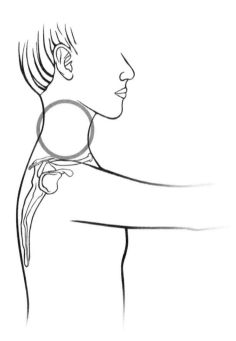

Ball Placement for the Side of the Neck

2. THE BACK OF THE HEAD

The fascia surrounding your skull is continuous with other soft tissue extending forward into your face, and down through your spine and legs. Working on the back of the head can help release this whole connected line, as well as relieve headaches and general stress. It might surprise you to find how much sensation is ready to be explored in the back of your head and how good it can feel!

Ball: One soft or medium 4″ ball

Body position: Lying on your back, possibly on a bolster or cushion to keep your spine neutral when the ball is under your head

Starting position of the ball: On the center of the back of your head

Action: After settling to release your head into the ball, begin to make very small and slow movements in any direction. Linger where you feel tightness.

Progression: Reposition the ball with your hand or by turning your head. Find any spot that is available, including the sides of the skull near the back of your ears. To reach the side, you can partially turn your body to one side.

Duration: 10 minutes

Contraindications: Extreme vertigo, recent concussion

Notes: This can be very relaxing, but I do not recommend falling asleep while practicing this technique!

Anatomy: Cranial fascia (galea aponeurotica), occipitalis muscle

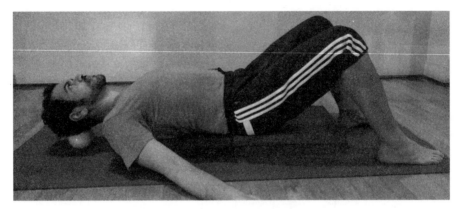

The Back of the Head

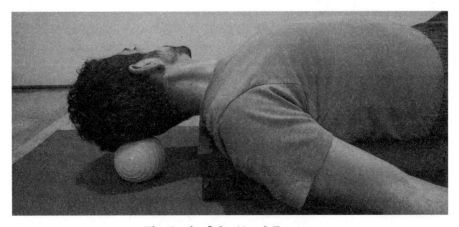

The Back of the Head, Turning

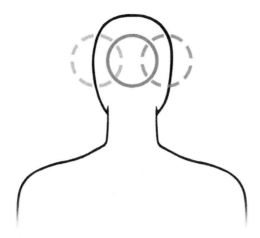

Ball Placement for the Back of the Head

3. THE TOP OF THE HEAD

As with the previous technique, there's more to explore here than you might expect. Our skull bones do move, and the gentle pressure of the ball here can encourage that healthy movement. The fascia covering your skull is connected to the fascia of your face and the fascia all the way down the back of your body. Most people find this technique to be gentle and very pleasant. You can control the pressure by your position and by the ball you choose, making it gentler or more vigorous as you wish. This technique can be done standing at a wall, on hands and knees on the floor, or while draping your body off the edge of a bed or couch.

Ball: One medium-sized hollow or solid ball, 3″, 4″, or 5″

Body position: There are three possible positions to try:

1. Standing near a wall

2. On your hands and knees with your head tucked down, bringing the top of your head to rest on the ball

3. Lying face down on the edge of a low bed or couch, curving your upper body down toward the floor to rest the top of your head on the ball.

Starting position of the ball: Touching the top of your head

Action: Slowly explore the top of your head with the ball. You may find some spots to be tender and others to have very little sensation.

Progression: Reposition the ball with your hand at any time. Explore the entire top of your head, moving slowly. Adjust the pressure by leaning more or leaning less onto the ball.

Duration: 5 minutes

Contraindications: Recent concussion

Anatomy: Cranial fascia (galea aponeurotica)

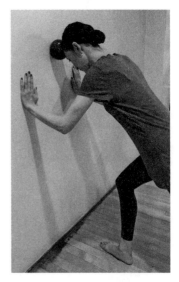

The Top of the Head

4. THE FACE

Stress often manifests as facial tension that can become so habitual that we take it for granted. Do you have wrinkles between your eyebrows from frowning or squinting? Do you hold your mouth a certain way when you are upset or angry? Do you grind your teeth? These tension patterns sneak up on us over years and literally reconfigure our facial expressions. Working on your face with the balls is a treat, and your family and friends may even comment on a subtle change in the way you look.

Ball: One small, fairly soft, hollow 2"–3" ball

Body position: Lie face down and support your body as needed. My suggestions for support: your mid-torso on a folded blanket or pillow, a blanket roll under your ankles, and a small pillow or rolled blanket under each shoulder. This will enable you to lie comfortably face down without strain in your neck, spine, shoulders, or legs.

Starting position of the ball: Under the center of your forehead

Action: Slowly roll your head to change the position of the ball very slightly. Your first movement might be turning your head very slowly from side to side, moving the ball horizontally across your forehead. Then you can nod your head to move the ball vertically up and down from the top to the bottom of your forehead. Or you can find a combination diagonal movement, or zigzag the ball across your forehead. Explore and spend time where you find tension.

Progression: Work across the middle of your forehead, then move the ball up and work across the upper forehead, then move the ball down to explore the lower forehead and eyebrows.

Progress down onto your jaw muscle and around the edge of your lower jaw. Open and close your mouth to feel the pressure and movement in your masseter muscle.

Explore across your cheeks, especially near the sides of your nose.

Finish your session with the ball in a place on your face that feels particularly good.

Duration: 5–10 minutes

Contraindications: Recent dental surgery or cosmetic facial surgery.

Notes: Remember to move slowly. If you are pregnant and cannot lie face down on the floor, you can sit in a chair with your knees wide apart, with a table for the ball to rest on.

Anatomy: All facial muscles: masseter, corrugator supercilii, temporalis, frontalis, procerus, zygomaticus major and minor, orbicularis oris, buccinator, risorius, platysma, depressor anguli oris, depressor labii inferioris, levator anguli oris, levator labii superioris, mentalis

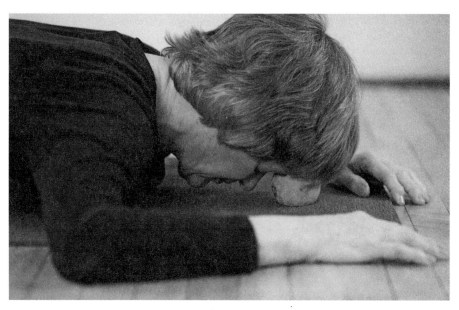

The Face

Denise, an administrator who spends too much time under pressure at the computer, was having pain in her jaw, numbness in her fingers, and chronic headaches. We worked with the ball on the side of her neck and her face for just one session. Her pain lessened, and she could clearly feel the connection between the tightness she carried and her symptoms. The ballwork has given her a convenient way to interrupt the usual pattern of tension buildup, and she has continued to be symptom-free.

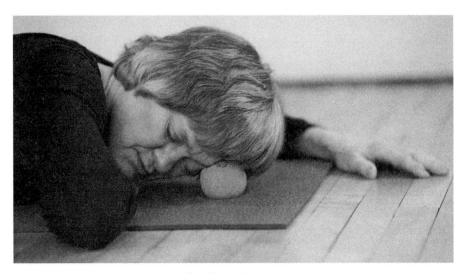

The Face, Turning

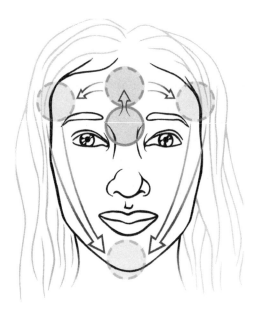

Ball Placement for the Face

CHAPTER 10

The Abdomen, Ribs, and Breathing

Although this area of the body may be sensitive, it is worthwhile working on because the results can yield tremendous opening in your spine and your breathing. It's an area of emotional holding and self-protection, so proceed at your own pace. Release here can increase your sense of groundedness and calm, connecting you to your center.

1. THE ABDOMEN, DIAPHRAGM, AND ILIOPSOAS

The title of this technique hints that these three muscular structures are very closely connected. The rectus abdominis, a superficial muscle, flexes the spine and can become short with excessive sitting or any exercise that involves spinal flexion, such as crunches or bicycling. When this muscle is shortened and tight, the diaphragm does not have the freedom to move down as we take a breath in. The iliopsoas attaches to the same part of the spine as the crura (tendons) of the diaphragm, making a functional link between hip flexion (walking or sitting) and breathing. Thus we work on them at the same time with the balls.

Balls: Two 4″ or 5″ hollow balls, optionally one football-shaped ball

Body position: Lie face down, with padding for your forehead if needed. If this is uncomfortable for any reason, you can work on these areas while standing near a wall.

Starting position of the balls: Begin with the balls under the fronts of your hips for a few minutes to settle. This addresses the lower end of the iliopsoas and gives space in the abdomen for the breath; it's an accessible way to begin.

Action: Once you have settled, begin to move your hips slowly to one side, then back to center, and then to the other side. Avoid pressing into the balls, but simply allow your body weight to provide the pressure.

Progression: When you are ready, move the balls up above your hip sockets, onto your lower abdomen. Work there for a few minutes, gently shifting from side to side.

Then remove one ball, and begin to slowly roll the remaining ball across your abdomen, staying longer in areas that feel tight. Follow a zigzag pathway to find all the different areas of the abdomen that you can reach with the ball. Move your body over the ball, and occasionally reposition the ball with your hand.

When the ball is near the anterior superior iliac spine (ASIS), you can perhaps feel the psoas as it joins the iliacus muscle.

When the ball is near the lower ribs, you will be as close as possible to the diaphragm muscle. Find places to work all along the lower edge of the ribs.

Duration: 10-15 minutes

Contraindications: Digestive problems, pregnancy, abdominal surgery. Those with irritable bowel syndrome can try a short amount of time on the balls and evaluate the results.

Notes: Try supporting your torso up on your forearms, in a "sphinx" position. This might provide more access to the upper abdomen, more freedom to breathe, and more weight while working on the lower abdomen.

The pathway of the large intestine goes up from the lower pelvis on the right side, then across the abdomen, then down on the left side. To help relieve constipation, follow that pathway with the ball.

The football-shaped ball works well with this abdomen technique.

Anatomy: Rectus abdominis, iliopsoas, iliacus, abdominal obliques, digestive and reproductive organs

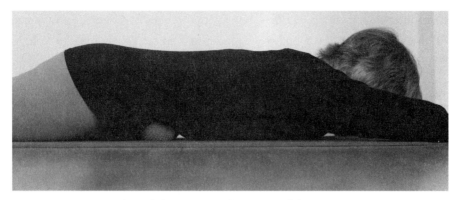

The Abdomen, Diaphragm, and Iliopsoas

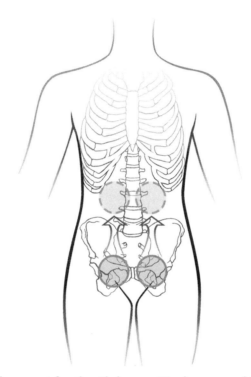

Ball Placement for the Abdomen, Diaphragm, and Iliopsoas

Martha is a dance teacher who has had tightness in her iliopsoas muscle for her whole career. "When I practice, I can feel my breath deepen and the tension in my body begin to release. For at least twenty years I have been a regular practitioner of this work, and practice at least twice a week. I love the freedom that the work provides. I travel with the balls and, despite a long trip or an unfamiliar bed, the ballwork is there like an old reliable friend to help ease any discomfort—or just to simply deepen the breath in an effort to let go after a long day."

2. THE SIDE WAIST / OBLIQUES

In addition to keeping good strength in the abdominals, we also benefit from maintaining length in the waistline area (meaning everything between the ribs and the pelvis), which is supported by the abdominal oblique muscles. We have two sets of abdominal oblique muscles (external and internal) wrapping around the waistline and connecting to the ribs, the fascia of the navel area, the fascia of the lumbar spine, and the pelvic rim. Their tone supports the lumbar spine and the abdominal organs, but excessive tightness here can hamper breathing, digestion, and lumbar mobility. Those who sit for many hours a day are prone to collapse and shortening in this area, and ballwork can reestablish spaciousness in this often forgotten part of the body.

Ball: One 4" or 5" ball, which can be soft, medium, or firm as you wish

Body position: Lying on your side, with adequate support for your head

Starting position of the ball: On the side waist, ideally free of the lower ribs and pelvic bones

Action: After an initial adjustment time to get used to the position and the pressure of the ball, do small movements forward and back. You can also turn slightly toward the floor, and then upward, to access different spots on the abdominal muscles.

Repeat on the other side.

Progression: If you have room to move the ball either up or down, you can find more areas to work with.

Duration: 5-10 minutes per side

Contraindications: Recent meal, recent abdominal surgery, intestinal irritability

Notes: Be sure to arrange the rest of your body comfortably with support for your head and possibly for your upper leg.

Anatomy: Digestive organs, internal oblique, external oblique, transversus abdominis, edge of quadratus lumborum

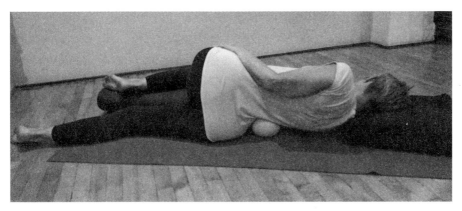

The Side Waist / Obliques

3. AROUND THE RIBS

Our ribs move constantly as we breathe—but how free are they for this move-ment? How easy is it for you to take a deep, satisfying breath? Do your ribs feel heavy and stiff, or light and mobile? It's amazing how quickly breath-ing difficulties can escalate into mental stress, and vice versa. The nervous system responds very quickly to changes in our breathing patterns. Shortness of breath is not a healthy condition, and yet we often don't notice it, or we may even assume it's our normal state. The ribs and lungs can lose their resil-iency from inactivity, emotional strain, fatigue, excessive coughing, or other respiratory illness. Ballwork for the ribs brings welcome relief.

Ball: One fairly soft 4″ ball

Body position: Lying on your side, with adequate support for your head

Starting position of the ball: On the spine, just below your shoulder blades

Action: After settling and breathing for a few minutes, begin to make very small movements in any direction. Move slowly, and explore both small side-to-side movements as well as small up-and-down movements. Each small, slow movement will reveal different sensations in your ribs and lungs, so take your time to feel the subtleties.

Progression: Progress around the entire rib cage, with these locations as stop-ping places: the right back side of the ribs, the right side of the ribs, and the right front side of the ribs. When you get to the center of the front, avoid the xiphoid process (the bottom of the sternum bone) but find a spot either above it on the sternum, or below it on the rectus abdominis muscle. Then continue around onto the left front ribs, the left side ribs, and the left back ribs. Finally, return to your starting place on the spine. When you remove the ball and lie flat, notice your breathing and overall state of being. You can also try some simple rib movements, such as the Cat-Cow movement of curving, arching, and circling the ribs and spine while on your hands and knees.

Duration: 15 minutes

Contraindications: Fractured rib, extreme respiratory distress, pleural infection or effusion

Notes: Rearrange your arms and legs in any way that's comfortable as you slowly progress around the ribs.

Anatomy: Intercostals, diaphragm, lungs, visceral and lung pleura and fascia

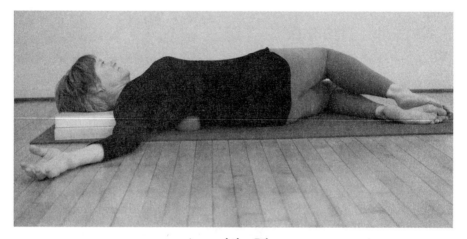

Around the Ribs

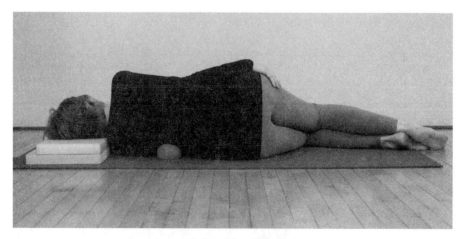

Around the Ribs, Side Lying

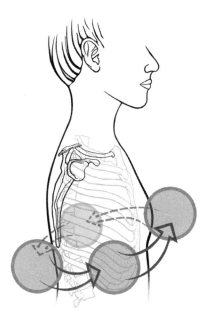

Ball Placement for Around the Ribs

4. THE STERNUM

Tension and constriction in the area of the sternum (breast bone) can result from breathing difficulties, emotional strain, shoulder strain, or rib subluxation. This technique will encourage easier movement in the sternum and its connection to the ribs. I recommend combining this technique with the balls on the upper spine and on the pectoralis muscle, which attaches to the sternum. (See the Front Chest with Two Balls, p 108.)

Ball: One medium-soft 4″, 5″, or 6″ ball or the football-shaped ball

Body position: Lying face down, with a small folded towel to support your forehead if you wish. An alternate position is standing against a wall.

Starting position of the ball: Against the middle of the sternum

Action: Spend a few minutes relaxing onto the ball, letting your upper back and chest drape around it. Determine if the ball is the right size and texture for you. Breathe mindfully, feeling the movement of the breath in your ribs and sternum. Then begin to move your sternum very carefully and slowly in any direction. You might start with a side-to-side movement, and then also try an up-and-down movement. While extending your chest forward, you can lift your head or use your arms for support if this feels good.

Progression: Move the ball higher on your sternum and do the same slow movement exploration. Then move the ball lower on the sternum, but not at the very bottom, because the xiphoid process is more delicate than the rest of the sternum. When you are finished, lie for a few minutes face down, then roll over onto your back and feel your breath, your spine, and anything else that might have changed.

Duration: 5–10 minutes

Contraindications: Sharp pain from rib subluxation (as opposed to a dull ache)

Notes: This technique can be quite intense or quite mild, so proceed at your own pace.

Anatomy: Sternum bone, ribs, intercostals, lungs, surrounding fascia

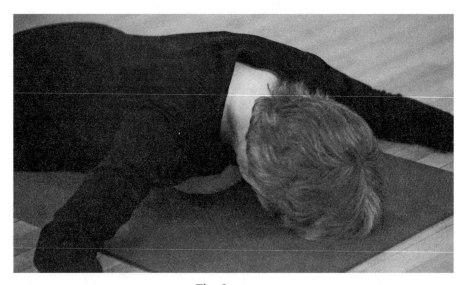

The Sternum

Judy, a health researcher, suffered a fall that caused sharp, stabbing pains in her ribs. After checking that there was no fracture, she started using the balls very carefully to explore what was happening in her soft tissue. She used a very soft 4" ball for a few minutes at a time, slowly coaxing the fascia and muscles to accept the pressure and become more adaptable. She worked around the rib cage little by little and was amazed at how quickly her pain subsided.

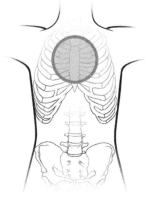

Ball Placement for the Sternum

CHAPTER 11

The Shoulders

Of all the areas of the body where students have found relief by using the balls, the shoulder area is at the top of the list. Our shoulders have a large range of motion with complex biomechanics that can easily go awry from too little or too much activity, poor alignment, or general stress. Nagging pain in the top or back of the shoulder, rotator cuff strain, general constriction and tightness—all of these symptoms are treatable and responsive to ballwork. The techniques in this chapter supplement the basic technique for the trapezius muscle that is outlined in chapter 7. Each technique targets muscles that restrict the free movement of the shoulder blades and contribute to poor posture. Students often say, "I feel that my shoulders finally fit onto my body the way they are supposed to" or "I never knew my shoulders could feel this loose."

Try each one, loosen your tight spots, and create a wonderful feeling of spaciousness and freedom.

1. ONE BALL FOR THE SHOULDER AND RIBS

The scapulae ride on the rib cage, moving in many directions to provide the large range of motion we have for arm movements. When the scapulae are held or restricted by muscle tension, the coordination of the entire "shoulder team" is disrupted, and compensations begin to accumulate. This ballwork technique helps to free the movement of the scapulae on the back ribs, as well as release rib tension. When the ribs are mobile, breathing is more satisfying.

Ball: One hollow 4″ or 5″ ball or the football-shaped ball

Body position: On your back, with a pillow or folded blanket ready to support your head, and possibly a bolster or larger cushion to support your arm when it stretches back next to your head.

Starting position of the ball: On the spine, between your shoulder blades

Action: This technique works on one side at a time, but we start in the center. First spend a few minutes breathing and releasing your weight into the ball. Feel the natural movement of your ribs and shoulders with each breath. Then begin to move your ribs and spine slowly and gently, in any direction that you can move.

Progression: Move the ball to one side of your spine, let's say to the right. Tilt your body slightly to the left, and rest your left shoulder on the floor. Support your head if needed. The ball will now be in the rhomboid area between your shoulder blade and your spine, on the right side, and your right shoulder will be off the floor. Rest your arms where they are most comfortable.

From here, there are three movement explorations in this first spot, with the same three explorations to follow in two other spots.

Movement 1: Move your shoulder blade in any direction it can move, very slowly, without lifting your arm. Concentrate the movement as close as possible to where the ball is touching.

Movement 2: Lift your right arm in the air and bend your elbow. With the arm lifted, you have a greater range of motion and more variety of pressure angles on the ball. Explore all possible movements of your arm in the air, very slowly and mindfully.

Movement 3: Stretch your arm next to your head, reaching back and touching the floor if possible. Use a folded blanket or bolster to support your hand if it does not easily rest on the floor. Breathe slowly and deeply, stretching longitudinally through the entire right side of your body, from your hand through your foot, while you inhale. Let your body settle back to a rest position as you exhale. Breathe rhythmically in this way several times.

Before moving the ball to a different spot, take it out from under you and feel the results. How is your breath? How are your ribs and shoulder blade on that side?

Then move the ball to a higher spot, still between your shoulder blade and your spine. Repeat all three movements here.

There is one more spot, lower than the first, near the lower end of your shoulder blade. Repeat the same series of three movements here, then remove the ball and feel the results. Compare your right and left chest and shoulder.

Now you have worked on one shoulder, and you can repeat the entire series on the other side.

Duration: 10 minutes per side

Contraindications: Recent muscle tear or rib subluxation

Notes: Choose a ball that feels comfortable but also gives you a good stretch. Spend more time in any area that feels tight or enjoyable, or both.

Anatomy: Ribs, intercostals, rhomboids, erector spinae, small muscles of the vertebral column (transversospinalis)

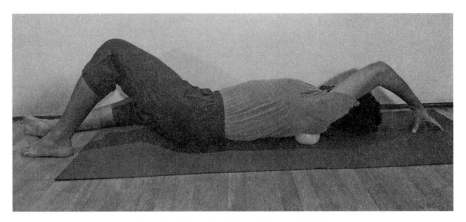

One Ball for the Shoulder and Ribs

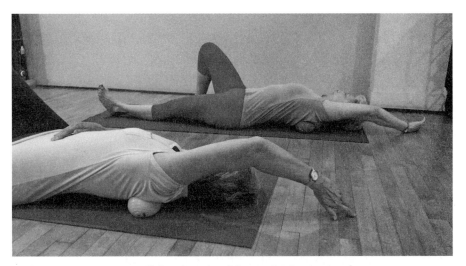

One Ball for the Shoulder and Ribs, Variation

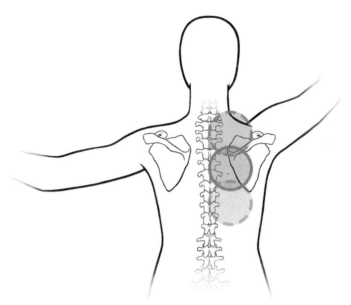

Ball Placement for One Ball for the Shoulder and Ribs

2. THE FRONT CHEST WITH TWO BALLS

This technique works with the pectoralis major and pectoralis minor muscles in the front upper chest. These muscles pull the shoulders forward, a very common misalignment that leads to reactive tightness in the back of the shoulders. Tension here can make your chest feel heavy and it can restrict your breath. This technique can help to relieve lung congestion.

In my studio we have affectionately nicknamed this technique "Kim's Bliss," after my student Kim, who found that it really helps her shoulders and upper back to stay open. She always starts her ballwork session with this one.

Balls: Two hollow 4" or 5" balls

Body position: Lying face down with optional small support for your forehead. If you have large breasts, you might like to have a folded blanket or cushion under your hips to help angle the upper chest properly on the balls.

Starting position of the balls: One under each side of the upper chest, above the breasts and below the collarbones, close to the center. Stretch your arms out to the sides with the palms down.

Action: Once you have taken time to settle and breathe, begin the first of three movements.

Movement 1: Slowly shrug your shoulders. Move minimally and notice sensations anywhere in the area of your shoulders.

Movement 2: Move your upper chest slowly to one side by reaching out through one arm at a time. The ball will roll across your pectoralis major muscle. Return to center, then roll to the other side slowly, then roll back to center.

Movement 3: Make a swimming movement with both arms, as in the breast stroke. Lifting your arms barely off the floor, bring them up toward your head, and then spread them out in a circular movement that brings them down by the sides of your body. Continue in this pattern several times, stopping along the way if you wish. When your arms are overhead, you can move your chest to each side slowly. When your arms are down by your sides, you can rotate your arms inward and then outward. Move very slowly.

Movement 4: Combine any of the above movements with a rotation of the arms, turning your palms up and down.

Progression: Move the balls farther apart. You will probably have room for three or four locations of the balls, each time repeating movements 1, 2, and 3. The last location for the balls can be on the tops of your arms, on the deltoid muscles. When finished, remove the balls and turn over onto your back to feel the results.

Duration: 15-20 minutes

Contraindications: Breast surgery

Notes: This technique is not especially intense with hollow balls, so if you want more pressure, use a harder ball or a solid ball.

If you have time, progress down the biceps and forearms with firm 4″ balls. See the instructions in chapter 12 for technique 3, Floor Balls for the Biceps, and technique 6, Floor Balls for the Lower Arms.

Anatomy: Pectoralis major, pectoralis minor, intercostals, deltoids

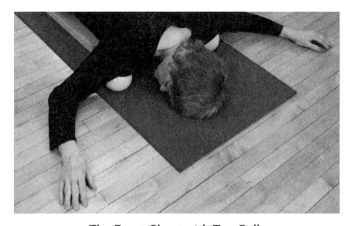

The Front Chest with Two Balls

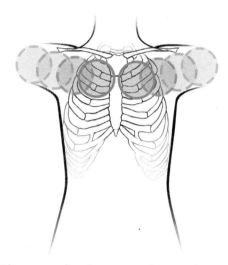

Ball Placement for the Front Chest with Two Balls

3. THE ROTATOR CUFF

The rotator cuff is a group of four muscles whose job is to secure the arm into the shoulder socket and to rotate it. Strain or tear in this team is a very common shoulder injury. The most common location of injury is the common tendon shared by three of the four muscles. This tendon is in the back of the shoulder joint, where the supraspinatus, the infraspinatus, and the teres minor all converge to attach to the humerus. Injury to this tendon frequently causes the deltoid muscle to spasm as it tries to take over the functions of the injured rotator cuff. Working with the balls can help to restore normal movement and reduce compensations. To reach the fourth muscle, subscapularis, use the Serratus Anterior technique (below).

Balls: Two medium-sized balls, 3"–4", hollow or solid according to your preference

Body position: Lying on your back, arms extended to the sides, perpendicular to your body axis

Starting position of the balls: One ball under each shoulder blade

Action: After a short time releasing into the balls and breathing, there are two movements:

Movement 1: Slowly shift your upper body to one side, allowing the ball to roll laterally across your shoulder blades. Return to center, and then slowly shift to the other side, again allowing the ball to roll laterally across your shoulder blades. Note any differences between the left and right sides.

Movement 2: Bend your elbows, bringing your hands to point upward toward the ceiling. Slowly rotate your upper arms, bringing the hands toward your feet (medial rotation of the humerus bone), with your palms pointing downward toward the floor. Slowly return to the starting position. Then rotate your upper arms in the other direction, bringing your hands back toward your head, with the backs of your hands toward the floor. This is lateral rotation of the humerus bone.

Progression: Reposition the balls wider apart to access a different section of the rotator cuff muscles. Repeat movements 1 and 2 in this new location.

Find more locations on the surface of your shoulder blades, and repeat the same movements.

Duration: 5-10 minutes

Contraindications: Extreme pain from recent injury

Notes: If you are tight, the range of motion will be small at first. Gradually work to increase your range.

Anatomy: Infraspinatus, teres minor

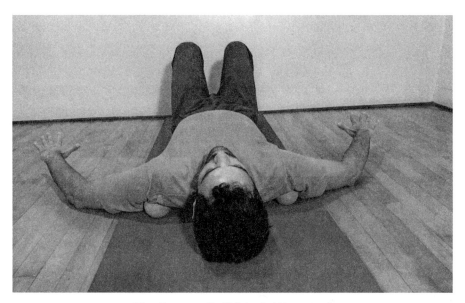

The Rotator Cuff (Medial Rotation)

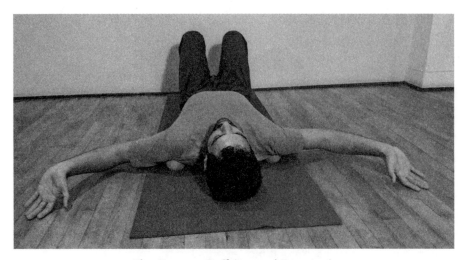

The Rotator Cuff (Lateral Rotation)

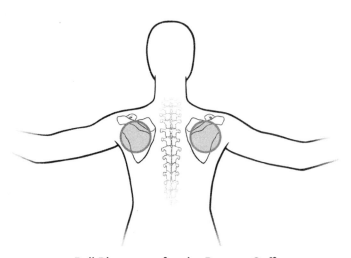

Ball Placement for the Rotator Cuff

4. WALL BALLS FOR THE PECTORALS AND DELTOIDS

With this technique, all you need is a space on the wall. No need for a sticky mat, a clear floor, or removing your shoes. You'll be standing up, working on one side at a time. Students find that this is a very convenient way to work on trigger points in the shoulder area and regain a feeling of spaciousness and freedom.

Balls: One 4″ hollow ball and one 2.5″ solid ball

Body position: Standing near a wall

Starting position of the ball: Stand facing the wall, and place the hollow ball on your sternum. With your feet close to the wall, the pressure will be less. Standing with your feet farther from the wall will create more pressure.

Action: Move the ball off to one side of your sternum. Press into the ball with your body weight to get the pressure that you want. Make very small movements around this first spot, such as moving side to side, then up and down (bending your knees).

Progression: After a few minutes on the first spot, move the ball farther toward your armpit. You will have three or four spots from the center out to your upper arm, contacting the pectoralis major and minor muscles. At any point, you can change to the solid ball if you want more pressure. You can also experiment with moving the arm on the same side, perhaps stretching it to the side against the wall and moving it upward.

Once you reach your upper arm, you may want to change to the solid ball for more pressure. The deltoid muscle is thicker and more fibrous than the pectoralis, so more pressure is appropriate. Work on three spots around the deltoid: front, side, and back.

Progress onto the surface of the scapula, on the rotator cuff muscles. Then finally work on the rhomboid, between the shoulder blade and the spine (not pictured).

Remove the ball and do some exploratory movements with both shoulders. Do they feel different? What changes can you feel in the side you worked with?

Repeat the same sequence on the other side: pectoralis major and minor, deltoid, rotator cuff, and rhomboids, working your way slowly around the shoulder.

Duration: 10-15 minutes per side

Contraindications: Recent shoulder surgery

Notes: Find the trigger points and give them more time.

Anatomy: Pectoralis major, pectoralis minor, deltoid, infraspinatus, teres minor, rhomboids, middle trapezius

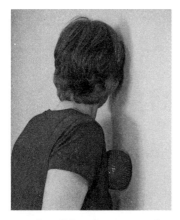

Wall Ball for the Pectorals

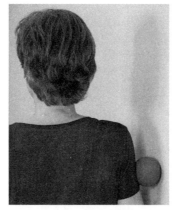

Wall Ball for the Deltoids

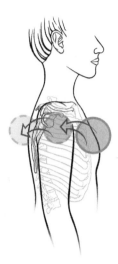

Ball Placement for the Wall Ball

5. SERRATUS ANTERIOR

This muscle lies partly under the shoulder blades, attaching to the medial border near the spine, and then wraps around to fan out onto the front surface of eight or nine ribs. Its job is to abduct the scapula, bringing it away from the spine, in opposition to the rhomboids, which pull the scapula toward the spine. Serratus anterior is well developed in body builders, but we all use it to hug each other or to fistfight, to do push-ups and yoga poses with our weight on the hands, or to carry heavy loads in front of us.

Chronic tightness in the serratus anterior can lead to round-shouldered posture, and compensatory tension (read: trigger point pain) in the trapezius and rhomboids. In the interest of balance, it's wise to work on all the muscles that move the scapulae, allowing them to work well as a team. This muscle is easily missed when the trapezius calls out for our attention so strongly.

Ball: One 4″ or 5″ ball, hard or soft according to your preference

Body position: Lying on your side with a block handy to support your head. If you're on your right side, your right arm stretches up beside your head to expose the armpit area. Rest your head on the block in front of your arm.

Starting position of the ball: Under the armpit area, placed so it can pull the shoulder blade back

Action: Settle into the position and feel the initial effects of the ball's pressure. How does it feel on your ribs? Shoulder? Neck? Can you arrange your arms comfortably? Make adjustments as needed.

When you are ready to move, shift slowly forward and back over the ball. See if you can catch the lateral edge of the shoulder blade and drag it back as the ball rolls. This will stretch the serratus anterior muscle.

Progression: Find another spot higher or lower on your side ribs, and do the same slow movements in these additional locations. When you are on a higher spot, you'll also be on the deltoid; and when you are on a lower spot, you'll catch the edges of subscapularis, triceps, and latissimus dorsi.

Repeat on the other side.

Duration: 5–8 minutes per side

Contraindications: Recent rotator cuff or other shoulder injury that prevents you from lying in this position

Notes: Be sure to arrange your head in a way that does not strain your neck. Be creative.

Anatomy: Serratus anterior, intercostals, deltoid, subscapularis, triceps, latissimus dorsi

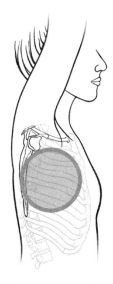

Ball Placement for the
Serratus Anterior

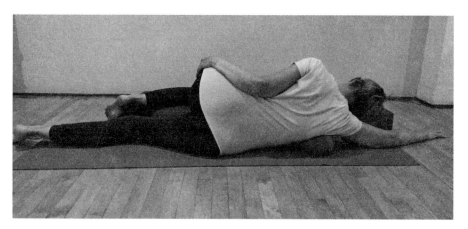

Serratus Anterior

CHAPTER 12

The Arms and Hands

How many different ways do you use your arms and hands in a typical day? Personal hygiene, cooking and eating meals, carrying a briefcase or a tote bag, working on a computer—all of these involve dexterity, which is a defining human trait. Perhaps you also do more specialized tasks like knitting, gardening, playing a musical instrument, drawing, or giving massages. If you're a yogi, you may stand on your hands or on your forearms. The hands and arms can accumulate extra tension and experience tissue restriction just like any other part of the body. Pain and tightness in the arms and hands can severely inhibit your daily activities, yet help is "at hand" with the balls. This chapter offers many ways to relieve sore spots and regain full use of your arms and hands. Some techniques are on the wall, some on the floor, and some sitting at a table.

Daniel is a musician whose primary instruments are keyboard and guitar. He came to me with spasms in his hands, which made playing very painful. We worked with the balls on his forearms and hands, and he reported that "it made a world of difference. I am so glad to have something I can do to release tension before, during, and after long sessions of playing. Just a few minutes does the trick."

1. WALL BALL FOR THE UPPER ARMS

If your shoulders need help releasing, it's likely that your upper arms do as well. There are three primary muscles here: the deltoids, which form the top contour of your shoulders and upper arms; the triceps at the back of your upper arm; and the biceps at the front. The fascia that surrounds these muscles can become torqued or matted together, causing movement restrictions and pain. This first technique is done standing against a wall, which means that you can do a few minutes of it at any time during your day—no need to change into exercise clothes or have a clear floor space to work in.

Ball: One firm ball, 2″, 3″, or 4″

Body position: Standing perpendicular to a wall with one shoulder against it

Starting position of the ball: Begin working on the deltoid, which has three sections: front, side, and back. You can start anywhere on the muscle.

Action: Establish the degree of pressure you want by leaning into the ball. Take a moment to slow down and feel your arm and the ball's pressure.

Begin to move slowly, at first up and down, then side to side. For the up-and-down movement, bend and straighten your knees. For the side-to-side movement, you can turn your arm only, or you can turn your whole body.

Progression: After working on the deltoid for several minutes, progress to the triceps. Turn slightly away from the wall and move the ball onto the back of your upper arm. In the same way as before, alternate between a movement up and down, and a movement side to side. You can vary the pressure by bending your elbow, then moving the arm slowly in any direction.

To access the biceps muscle, turn to face the wall and extend your arm out to one side. Place the ball on your biceps muscle, turn slightly away from the ball, and make small, slow movements in any direction to access different parts of the muscle.

Repeat on the other arm.

Duration: 5-8 minutes per arm

Contraindications: Recent surgery, abrasion, bruise, or fracture

Notes: There is a seam of fascia between the triceps and biceps that is worth working on as well. It will feel different—more tough and stringy, less bulky.

On the inner line of your upper arm, the blood vessels and nerves are near the surface, which will make this area quite tender. Stay on the muscles.

Anatomy: Deltoid, triceps, biceps, brachialis, intramuscular septum

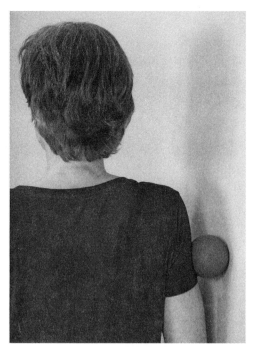

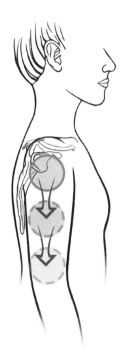

Wall Ball for the Upper Arm

Ball Placement for Wall Ball
for the Upper Arm

2. WALL BALL FOR THE LOWER ARMS

My students use this to relieve fatigue and tension in the wrists and hands, especially from typing. Racket sports enthusiasts can also benefit. The forearm muscles rarely get to stretch in daily life, so trigger points can easily develop and cause discomfort and wrist strain. A few minutes on the ball can make a huge difference. Like the upper arm technique above, there's no need to get onto the floor or change into exercise clothes—you can do a few minutes anywhere there is space on a wall.

Ball: One firm ball, 2″, 3″, or 4″

Body position: Standing facing the wall with your elbow bent and your forearm laterally placed across your front waist

Starting position of the ball: Start near your elbow, where there is thicker muscle tissue to work with. Place the ball between your forearm and the wall.

Action: To find the right pressure, lean into the ball as little or as much as you want. Begin a slow process of working the ball into the forearm extensor muscles. You can move the ball along the direction of the muscle's fibers, separating the bundles, or you can cross-friction the muscle by bending your knees. You will probably find some spots to be much more sensitive than others.

Progression: Patiently work through the entire outer forearm, from elbow to wrist.

Variation: Rotate your forearm, turning the palm of your hand up and down, which supinates and pronates your forearm.

To access the flexor muscles, turn around with your back to the wall, bend your elbow, and place your forearm along your back waist, with the palm facing the wall. Work through the entire forearm in the same way as before.

Repeat with the other arm.

Duration: 5–8 minutes per arm

Contraindications: Bruises or other recent injury

Notes: Don't be deterred by sensitive spots. You can always reduce the pressure by leaning away from the wall with your whole body. Be careful to maintain a slow speed.

Anatomy: Brachioradialis, extensor carpi radialis longus and brevis, extensor carpi ulnaris, extensor digitorum, flexor carpi radialis, flexor carpi ulnaris, palmaris longus, flexor digitorum superficialis and profundus, pronator teres, pronator quadratus, supinator

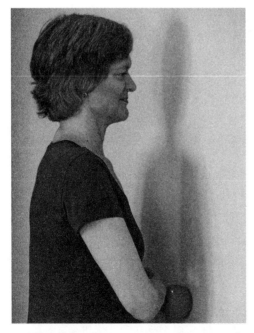

Wall Ball for the Lower Arm (Extensors)

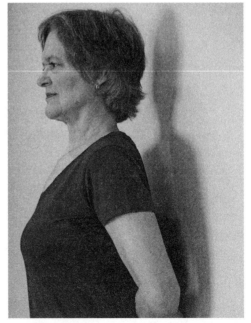

Wall Ball for the Lower Arm (Flexors)

3. FLOOR BALLS FOR THE BICEPS

The pressure you get from the balls in techniques 3-6 may be less than in the previous two techniques, because it comes from the weight of your arms rather than the weight of your body leaning into the wall. The trade-off is that you are lying down (more restful) and you can do both arms at once (more efficient). If you have two yoga mats, it is helpful to arrange them in a "T" shape so that your body has a vertical mat and your arms have a horizontal mat. This will help you to keep the balls where you want them.

Balls: Two firm 4″ or 5″ balls

Body position: Lying face down, arms to the sides, with a support for your head if you wish

Starting position of the balls: Under the proximal biceps muscles of each arm (near the shoulders)

Action: Take some time to settle, and be sure that the rest of your body is comfortable. You might want to put a small pillow under your chest, abdomen, or ankles.

Begin to move your arms very slowly. To move the ball along the fibers of the biceps, stretch one arm to the side, allowing your torso to move with it. This movement will bring the ball higher on one arm and lower on the other in a gliding motion. Then return to center. Move to the other side in the same way, slowly enough to feel each part of the biceps muscle. At any point, you can add a rotating motion, slowly turning your arm inward and then outward.

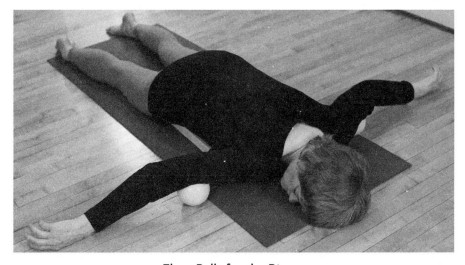

Floor Balls for the Biceps

Progression: Reposition the balls as needed, to work on the entire upper arm.

Duration: 5–10 minutes

Contraindications: Injury to the upper arm

Notes: It's easy to get going too fast, so make the effort to maintain a slow speed.

Anatomy: Biceps, brachialis

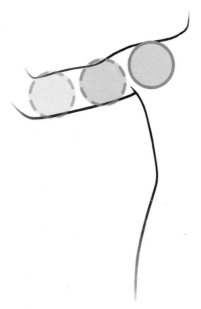

**Ball Placement for Floor Balls
for the Biceps**

4. FLOOR BALLS FOR THE TRICEPS

This technique is a good follow-up to any shoulder work, because the triceps muscle crosses both the elbow and the shoulder joints. It is also very good for elbow pain.

Balls: Two balls of equal size and texture, 3″–4″ according to your preference

Body position: Lying on your back with your arms reaching out to each side

Starting position of the balls: On the back of the upper arms, near the shoulders

Action: Release the weight of your arms into the balls and breathe. Then move your upper body to one side in a gliding motion, keeping the weight on both balls if you can. Follow that with the same movement to the other side. This moves the balls along the direction of the fibers of the triceps muscle.

This side-to-side movement can be done with your elbows straight or bent. You can also cross-friction the muscle by turning your arms inward and then outward, with your elbows bent.

Progression: Reposition the balls as needed to work on the entire upper arm.

Duration: 5-10 minutes

Contraindications: Recent injury

Notes: Don't worry if the left and right balls are not on the same area of each arm.

Anatomy: Triceps

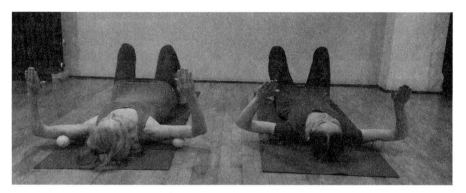

Floor Balls for the Triceps

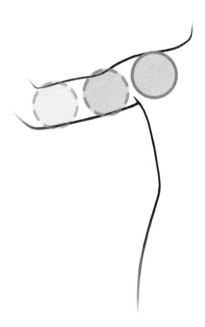

**Ball Placement for Floor Balls
for the Triceps**

5. CHAIR OR TABLE BALL FOR THE TRICEPS

This technique highlights the back of the upper arm, and its connection into the shoulder and the back. Tension here can make it difficult or impossible to bring your arms overhead, which is required by many yoga poses and by daily tasks such as putting on a shirt, replacing a light bulb, or reaching up to a high shelf.

Ball: One firm 3″–4″ ball

Body position: Two choices: (1) sitting at a table or (2) sitting on the floor next to a chair or bench as shown here.

Starting position of the ball: At the top of your upper arm, near your shoulder

Action: Fold your elbow and place the ball under your triceps muscle at the back of your upper arm. To create some pressure, lean into it as much as you want. Then move slowly in any direction over one spot at a time. You can move slowly along the arm, following the direction of the fibers of the muscle as you extend the elbow out away from you. You can also cross-friction the muscle by rotating

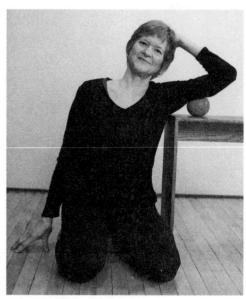

Chair or Table Ball for the Triceps

your arm forward as if to put your palm down, then moving the other way, tilting your hand back. The ball will move across the fibers of the muscle, helping to loosen tension.

Progression: Move the ball incrementally along your upper arm, anywhere between your shoulder and your elbow. Work in the same slow way in each spot.

Repeat with the other arm.

Duration: 5–10 minutes per arm

Contraindications: Recent injury

Notes: Be sure that the rest of your body is comfortable. If you do this technique on the floor, sit with your hips on a support to avoid lower back or hip strain.

Anatomy: Triceps, latissimus dorsi, shoulder capsule

6. FLOOR BALLS FOR THE LOWER ARMS

I recommend that you work on both sides of the lower arms, regardless of where your discomfort is. This description begins with the wrist and finger flexors while lying face down, and then continues onto the wrist and finger extensors while lying on your side.

Balls: Two firm balls of equal size and texture, 2″–4″

Body position: Lying face down at first, arms out to the sides. Use extra support under your hips, chest, or forehead if needed.

Starting position of the balls: Under the upper part of each inner forearm, the proximal flexor muscles

Action: Begin by settling, and releasing the full weight of your arms onto the balls.

Check that the rest of your body has adequate support, and add cushioning where needed. Then begin to move slowly, in any direction that allows the balls to access the flexor muscles. You can extend your arms out away from you, moving the balls along the fiber direction of the muscles, or you can cross-friction by rotating your forearms.

Progression: Move the balls to different spots along your entire forearms. Spend more time in the areas that feel tight.

When you are finished with the flexors, roll over onto your right side, adding some support under your head and under your ribs. Place your right forearm on the balls, and add the weight of your left forearm over the right one. Then slowly move the entire forearm over the balls, accessing the wrist and finger extensors. You can move the balls along the fiber direction of the muscles (toward your hands, toward your elbow), or you can cross-friction the balls by rotating your forearm.

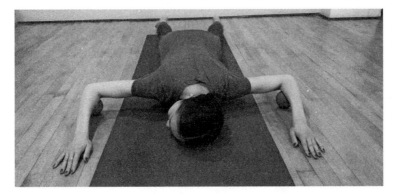

Floor Balls for the Lower Arms (Lying Prone for Flexors)

Repeat on the left forearm.

Duration: 5-10 minutes for the flexors, 5-10 minutes for the extensors

Contraindications: Abrasions or other wounds on your arms

Notes: It is easy to start moving very fast, so remind yourself to slow down.

Anatomy: All wrist flexors and extensors, flexor digitorum and extensor digitorum

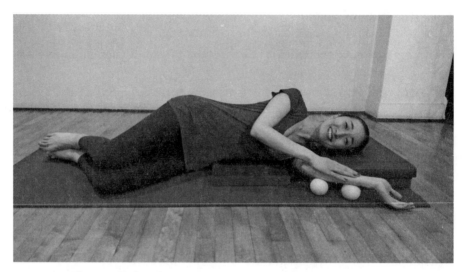

Floor Balls for the Lower Arms (Side Lying for Extensors)

7. TABLE BALL FOR THE LOWER ARMS

This technique is very useful for working on specific knots and trigger points in your forearms. For those who spend many hours typing, it's a perfect way to utilize your (hopefully) frequent breaks.

Ball: One 2.5″ ball

Body position: Sitting with your forearm resting on a table or desk

Starting position of the ball: Under any part of your forearm

Action: With one forearm on the desk, palm down, place your other hand on top of it to add more weight. Move slowly, rolling the ball toward the elbow and toward the wrist, or crisscrossing over the muscles by rotating your palm and forearm up and down very slowly. You can access both the flexors and extensors because of this rotation.

Progression: Find any sore or tight spots as you explore the length of your forearm.

Repeat with the other arm.

Duration: 5-10 minutes per arm

Contraindications: Bruises or other recent injury to your forearms

Notes: It is easy to start moving very fast, so remind yourself to slow down.

Anatomy: All wrist flexors and extensors, flexor digitorum and extensor digitorum

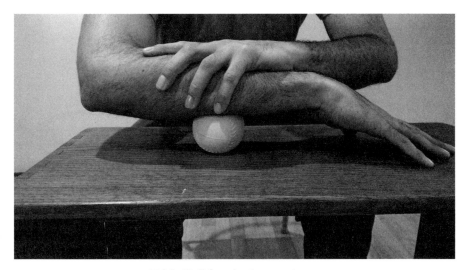

Table Ball for the Lower Arms

8. THE ARM NUTCRACKER

As with a similar technique for the legs (technique 7, The Leg Nutcracker, in chapter 14), you can control the intensity of this one. The ball will massage both the upper and lower arms simultaneously. You'll work on one arm at a time.

Ball: One 2.5″ ball of any texture

Body position: Standing near a wall

Starting position of the ball: Bend your elbow and place the ball between your lower and upper arm, then rest that forearm against the wall. Your other hand touches the ball to keep it from escaping.

Action: Slowly move from side to side, guiding the ball with your movement and with your free hand.

Progression: Move the ball to other spots and do the same slow movement.

Repeat with the other arm.

Duration: 5 minutes per arm

Contraindications: Recent injury

Notes: These muscles may be very rope-like, so the support of the second hand is very helpful to keep the ball in place and the movement as smooth as possible.

Anatomy: Biceps, wrist flexors

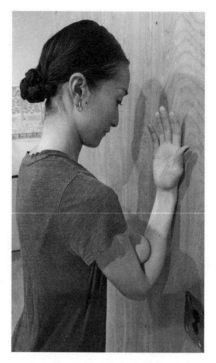

The Arm Nutcracker

9. HANDS ON THE TABLE OR FLOOR

You might be surprised at how much tension is held in your hands. That tension can be a result of your activities, or a result of arthritic changes in the finger joints that limit your movements. The fascia surrounding the muscles can become tight if we don't work to keep it resilient. This technique is especially good for yogis, musicians, carpenters, and massage therapists.

Ball: One small 1″–2″ ball of any texture

Body position: Sitting on the floor or near a table or desk

Starting position of the ball: Under the center of your palm

Action: Press down into the ball, and use your other hand to add pressure if you wish. Start with a slow circular movement, exploring the center of your palm.

Progression: Slowly progress to the mound of your thumb, out onto the thumb, and back to the palm again. Take extra time in the web between your thumb and index finger. Then work on the entire length of each finger, and the web between each finger. Proceed down the outer edge of the hand, and across the wrist. Spend extra time wherever you feel tension or stiffness.

Repeat on the other hand.

Duration: 5 minutes per hand

Contraindications: Recent injury

Notes: For a quick fix, rub one ball between your two hands with a kneading motion. Find any tight or sore spots, and roll them to relaxation.

Anatomy: Thenar group (muscles of the thumb) and hypothenar group (muscles of the pinky finger) muscles, palmar interossei, lumbricals

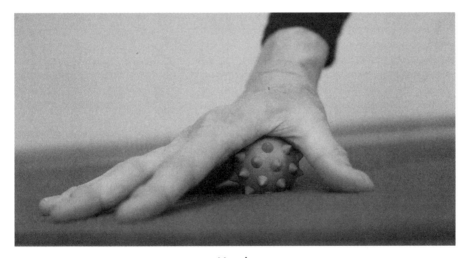

Hands

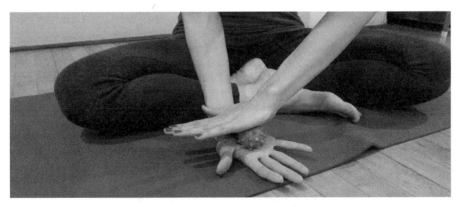

Two-Hand Variation

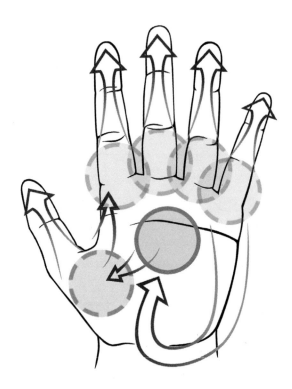

Ball Placement for Hands

Johanna is a piano teacher who developed trigger finger, a condition in which nodules form on the finger tendons and don't allow the finger to bend and straighten smoothly. She did the usual medical treatment—a cortisone shot—which helped for three months, but then the problem returned. Her doctor recommended surgery, but she wanted to try other things first. She tried acupuncture, massage, and skin creams, which all helped. Then she started working with a small ball on her hand, and she found that she could get into the tight spots very specifically. As a result of this targeted massage, the nodule shrank enough so that it is no longer a problem. She says, "I love the ballwork because I am in control—I can do what I can tolerate without fear. My participation in the process is the best thing. When I give it my full attention, it really works. In fact, I can truthfully say that the ballwork is the most successful self-care thing that I do."

CHAPTER 13

The Pelvis, Thighs, and Knees

As two-legged creatures, we are dependent on our hips and knees to walk, run, and jump. We swing one leg forward then the other, propel ourselves, catch ourselves, and readjust our balance constantly throughout the day, without thinking about it. The pelvis is the link between the upper and lower body, and mediates all of this locomotion. If we are healthy, these rather complex movements continue without much fuss or bother. If there is imbalance and strain, the simplest movements are painful, and life becomes restricted. One common situation with the large thigh and hip muscles is a constriction between layers; the fascia between the muscles becomes stuck and interrupts the smooth flow of each muscle's range of motion. The balls can help to free up this movement between the muscles.

The techniques in this chapter supplement the two hip techniques in chapter 7 (The Back of the Pelvis and The Front of the Hips) and give you many ways to target tight spots in your pelvis and upper legs for more freedom and ease. In addition to helping you move more easily, working on your legs will calm your nervous system, helping to move the prana downward through the legs. Try these techniques if you have a vata imbalance or if you travel frequently—they are great for jet lag.

Allison is a professional dancer who came to me with a complaint of intense pain in her thighs and hips from hamstring strain. Sitting on the balls helped her to release the bellies of the hamstring muscles and separate the big thigh muscles from being "glued" together. This took pressure off the hamstring tendons and allowed them to heal. It took only a few sessions for her to feel significant relief, and now she uses the balls regularly to avoid future injuries.

1. SITTING ON THE BALLS

Like the shoulders, the hips are complex structures with many layers of muscles and fascia and a wide range of motion. In the ideal world, if we could move the pelvis and hips in all directions evenly every day, the tone in the soft tissue in this area would be even, and the discomforts few. But that's not the way it works for many of us, who sit for hours every day. At the other end of the spectrum are those who practice yoga, martial arts, or dance, requiring greater-than-normal range of motion.

Deep tightness can develop below the surface and have adverse effects on our alignment and movements. This technique gets to the deepest layers of hip muscles and can give you a sense of freedom relatively quickly. I practice a variation of this one in airplanes, buses, and cars.

Balls: Two firm 3"–4" balls (hollow or solid)

Body position: Sitting on the floor, cross-legged at first. If this is difficult, you can try this technique sitting in a chair.

Starting position of the balls: Under the area near the sitting bones (the balls could be wider apart or closer together as you wish)

Action: Sitting up tall, notice the sensation of pressure in your buttocks muscles from the balls and your body weight. Then begin to move very slowly in any direction, exploring the deep hip muscles with the balls.

Progression: There are four ways to work:

1. Explore the pelvic fascia and muscles near your sitting bones. Move slowly in any direction, taking time if you find sore spots.

2. To reach the outer thighs: Bend one knee, and turn your body toward that leg. You'll have more weight on that leg, less on the other one. As you turn, the ball will progress into the outer hip. Find small, slow movements to explore a series of spots, progressing from your hip toward the knee. You can lean over the leg and press with your hands to create more pressure if you wish. Repeat on the other leg.

3. To reach the hamstrings: Extend both legs straight out in front of you with a bolster on top of your thighs to add more weight. Move your legs over the balls by slowly turning your legs inward and then outward.

Roll the balls incrementally down the backs of your legs. At each spot, turn your legs in and out to reach the inner and outer hamstring muscles. Progress from the hips down to the knees.

4. Sit on a firm chair with the balls under your hips, and move slowly to work into the muscles of the hips and thighs. Progress down toward your knees as far as possible.

Duration: 5-15 minutes
Contraindications: Movement restriction or injury (such as hamstring tendon tear) in the hip preventing you from being in this seated position
Anatomy: Gluteus maximus, gluteus medius, piriformis, gemellus inferior and superior, quadratus femoris, obturator externus and internus, iliotibial band, hamstrings, vastus lateralis

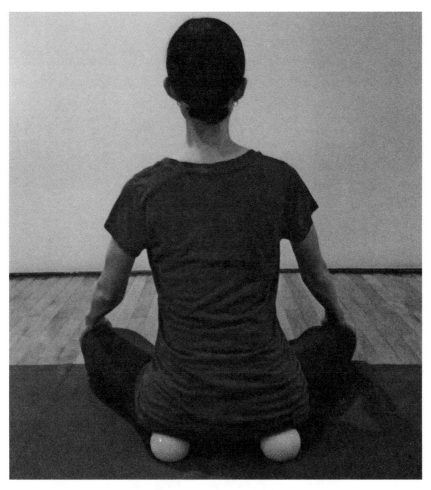

Sitting on the Balls 1

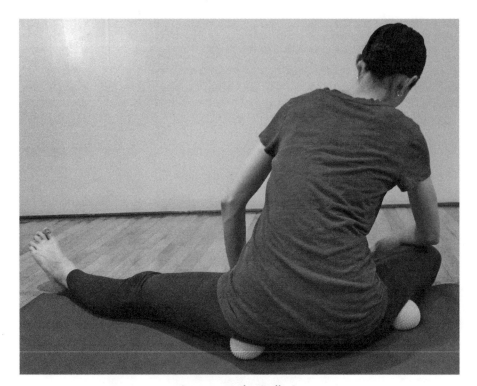

Sitting on the Balls 2

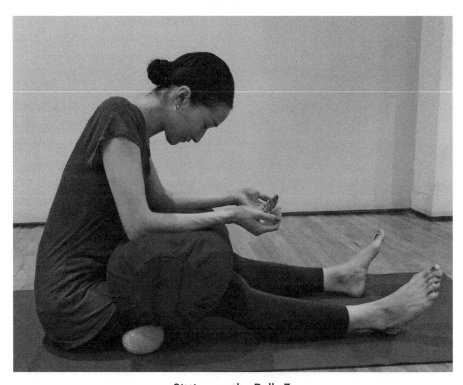

Sitting on the Balls 3

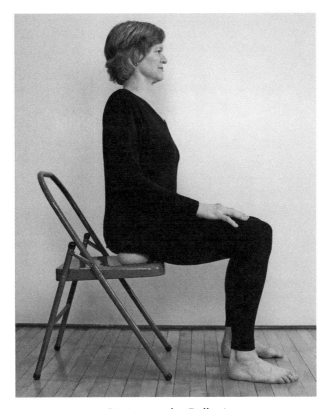

Sitting on the Balls 4

2. THE HAMSTRINGS LYING ON THE FLOOR

This technique is a gentler approach to working on the hamstrings, and you can do both legs at once while lying down. It's a wonderful thing to do at the end of a long day on your feet, and you can do it in bed as you prepare for sleep.

Balls: Two firm 5″ balls

Body position: Lying on your back

Starting position of the balls: Near the tops of the backs of your thighs. Find your "home base" position for the balls in which your legs can relax. That position might be with your legs turned out, or neutral, or turned in; it doesn't matter.

Action: Very slowly and gently, turn your legs inward toward the midline, then back to home base, then outward, then back to home base.

Progression: Gradually move the balls down farther on your legs, toward your knees. Work each spot slowly and carefully.

Duration: 10 minutes

Contraindications: None

Notes: If you want deeper pressure, you can place a folded blanket across your thighs. At first this technique may feel quite mild, but with time you will access deeper layers.

Anatomy: Biceps femoris, semitendinosus, semimembranosus

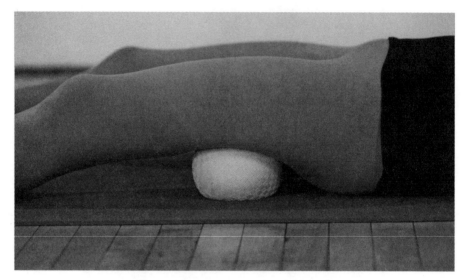

The Hamstrings Lying on the Floor

3. THE FRONT THIGHS

On the front of the thighs we have one large group of four muscles called the quadriceps whose main job is to straighten our knees. One of them (rectus femoris) crosses both the hip and the knee joints, but the others begin on the thighbone and only cross the knee. All four of them join together to form the large tendon that encircles the patella and then attaches to the tibia below the knee. These muscles can become overworked from lifting heavy objects, bicycling or hiking, any sport or dance that involves running and jumping, and of course, vigorous yoga. Chronic tightness in the quads can cause hip or knee pain, as well as misalignment of the entire lower leg. This technique can be intense at first, but quite soon the muscles learn to relax by working with the balls. As with all the leg techniques, releasing the thighs brings a generalized bodymind ease, and we feel more grounded.

Balls: Two 3″-5″ balls, either hollow or solid, according to your preference

Body position: Lying face down with a cushion or blanket under your torso to prevent hyperlordosis (overarching) of the lumbar spine and discomfort in the neck. You might also want a small support under your forehead and each shoulder. You can also support your ankles on a bolster.

Starting position of the balls: At the top of the thighs. Find a "home base" position for your legs in which you can relax. It might be in neutral rotation (knees facing down) or a light rotation inward or outward.

Action: There are three movements to try:

1. Very slowly roll your thighs in toward the midline, then back to the home base position, then outward away from the midline, and back to home base. This will cross-friction the quadriceps.

2. Bend your knees and do the same rotation, moving your foot and lower leg side to side very slowly. This position will create a deeper sensation, with more weight and a bit of stretch to the muscles.

3. Slowly elongate one leg at a time. This glides the ball over the muscle longitudinally and helps the muscles to slide over each other freely. You can do this with the leg bent or straight; try it both ways.

Progression: You can move both legs at once, or alternate legs to enable you to feel more detail. Gradually move the balls down your thighs, almost to the knee joints. When the muscles narrow to morph into the patellar tendon, you're at the stopping point.

Duration: 10 minutes

Contraindications: Difficulty lying face down, recent knee injury or surgery

Notes: Be sure that the rest of your body is comfortable. It doesn't make sense to work on your thighs but endanger your shoulders, neck, or lower back! Try coming up onto your forearms in a "sphinx" position for a change.

Anatomy: Rectus femoris, vastus medialis, vastus lateralis, vastus intermedius

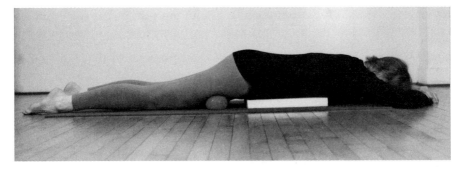

The Front Thighs 1

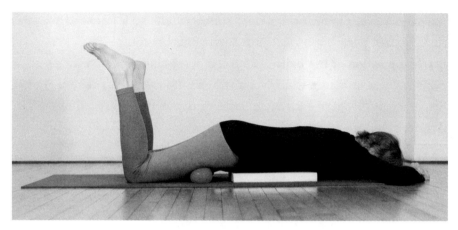

The Front Thighs 2

4. THE OUTER THIGHS

The iliotibial band (ITB) is now recognized by exercise enthusiasts as a locus of tightness and restriction in the hips and legs. The ITB runs from the iliac crest (top side rim of the pelvis) all the way down the outer thigh to attach below the outer knee. This strong band of connective tissue is crucial to our balance and coordination in walking and running, and we need it for that. However, the fascia and the muscles under it (vastus lateralis, one of the quadriceps) and above it (tensor fascia lata) can hold excess tension that may impact the hip and the knee. Layers of tissue that are meant to slide over each other become stuck together, causing constriction. Try this technique as an alternative to the foam roller to increase freedom in your hips and knees. You'll notice a new fluidity in your normal walking.

Ball: One or two 4″ balls, either hollow or solid

Body position: Lying on your side, legs bent, with the following supports: a folded blanket or pad under your side ribs (from waist to armpit), a higher support under your head to bring it level with the rest of your spine, and an optional bolster for your upper leg. There is a space between the rib support and head support, and that's where your shoulder rests. Without these supports, lying on your side can compress your shoulder and strain your neck.

Starting position of the ball: Under the upper part of the ITB, just below the upper rim of the pelvis. There is space for one ball between the upper rim of the pelvis and the greater trochanter, the bony prominence at the side of your hip.

Action: After settling, make small, slow movements with your pelvis. You can flex your hip, bringing your knee toward your chest. You might turn your pelvis toward or away from the floor, or move it forward and backward.

Progression: Avoiding the greater trochanter of the femur, move the ball down onto the side of your thigh. If you want to spread the pressure over a bigger area, making it less intense, add a second ball in line with the first one. As you work through each spot along your outer thigh to just above the knee, try these movements:

1. Move your leg forward and back.

2. Lift your foot off the floor, which will rotate the hip joint and create more pressure on the ball as it cross-frictions the muscle and fascia.

3. Explore the difference between working with your other leg in front of you or behind you; it will change the angle and degree of pressure of the ball. You can also add more weight by placing the top leg over the bottom leg.

Repeat on the other leg.

Duration: 10 minutes per leg

Contraindications: Recent hip surgery or injury

Notes: Because this is an intense technique, try it for just a few minutes at first.

Anatomy: Iliotibial band, tensor fascia lata, vastus lateralis

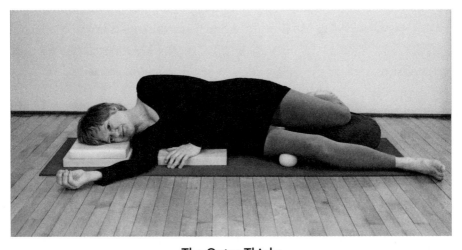

The Outer Thighs

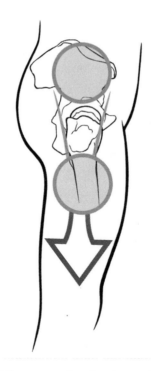

Ball Placement for the Outer Thighs

5. THE INNER THIGHS IN A CHAIR

The inner thigh muscles are the adductors, and they are major stabilizers in standing and walking. They can become tight and short over time if we don't stretch them, or if we are under chronic stress. This is the place to work if you have groin pain. There are two options: in a chair or on the floor. The chair version is good to use if your tension is closer to your hip, and the floor version is good to use if your tension is nearer the knee. You'll need a chair without arms, such as a folding chair or a bench, because you will sit with one leg on each side of the chair.

Ball: One large 5″ hollow ball

Body position: Sitting straddled on a chair with one leg bent to one side, the other leg behind you on the other side of the chair. Turn toward the bent leg.

Starting position of the ball: Under the top of your inner thigh on the back leg

Action: Once you have settled in a position that is workable for your hips, begin to make very small movements in any direction, allowing the ball to massage the top of your adductor muscles. Roll forward on your thigh by shifting your hips slightly back, and then roll to the back of the groin as you lean your upper body back and shift your hips forward.

Progression: Move the ball incrementally down your thigh as far as possible. Repeat on the other leg.

Duration: 5-8 minutes per leg

Contraindications: Inability to sit straddling the chair

Notes: If some spots are too sensitive to work with, pass over them briefly and work on nearby spots.

Anatomy: Gracilis, sartorius, pectineus, adductor brevis, adductor longus, adductor magnus, semitendinosus, semimembranosus

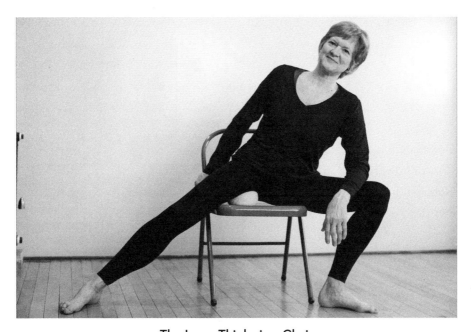

The Inner Thighs in a Chair

6. THE INNER THIGHS ON THE FLOOR

Working on the floor may require a bit more agility than working in a chair. The advantage is that with a comfortable setup, it's easier to spend more time when you're on the floor.

Ball: One large 5″-6″ ball

Body position: Lying on your side, legs bent, with the following supports: a folded blanket or pad under your side ribs (from waist to armpit) and a higher support under your head to bring it level with the rest of your spine. There is a space between the rib support and head support for your shoulder. Without these supports, lying on your side can compress your shoulder and strain your neck. You'll also need a block or a folded blanket to put under the ball.

Starting position of the ball: Stack the ball on top of the block, and bring the ball as high on your inner thigh as possible toward the groin. Roll slightly forward to get some weight on the ball. Your foot can rest on the floor.

Action: Try several different movements, which are small enough to keep the ball on the block:

1. Glide your leg away from you and back toward you very slowly, letting the ball massage along the direction of the muscle fibers.

2. Bend your leg up toward your chest, then down away from your chest.

3. Rotate the entire leg, lifting your foot off the floor.

Progression: Move the ball incrementally down your thigh to just above the knee and repeat the same actions.

Repeat on the other leg.

Duration: 5-10 minutes per leg

Contraindications: Extreme tenderness or a tear to an adductor muscle

Notes: You can vary the intensity easily by using a softer or firmer ball. You can also try it with two balls (and a block to support each one), spreading the pressure over a wider area.

Anatomy: Gracilis, sartorius, pectineus, adductor brevis, adductor longus, adductor magnus, semitendinosus, semimembranosus

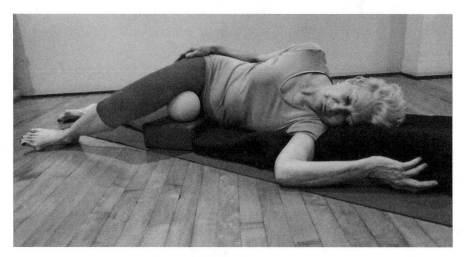

The Inner Thighs on the Floor

7. THE BACKS OF THE KNEES

This is one of the gentler ballwork techniques, because the knees bend easily and are not very heavy. It's a soothing thing to do if you've been on your feet all day. The ball gently separates the thigh and the shin bones, opening up the joint space and softening the back of the knee.

Balls: Two firm 5″ balls

Body position: Lying on your back

Starting position of the balls: Under the center of each knee

Action: First release, breathe, and find your "home base" position. Your legs may naturally want to turn out or turn in; let that happen. Your home base position is where your legs feel stable on the balls.

Progression: Slowly rotate your thighs inward, then back to home base, then outward, and back to home base again. Do this several times, stopping in places that feel like they need more time.

When you have done enough on this first spot, move the balls slightly higher to reach the lower end of the hamstring muscles. Work in the same way here, slowly turning your legs in and out.

Then move the balls slightly below your knees, onto the upper gastrocnemius. Do the same slow rotation here.

Duration: 10 minutes

Contraindications: Sharp pain in the knees

Notes: To create more pressure, place a block on either side of your knee and rest a blanket or sandbag over the knee, supported by the two blocks.

Anatomy: Knee capsule, tendons of hamstrings and gastrocnemius, plantaris and popliteus muscles, indirectly the bursae, menisci, and collateral and cruciate ligaments of the knees

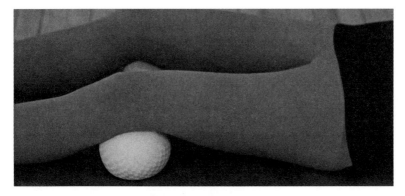

The Backs of the Knees

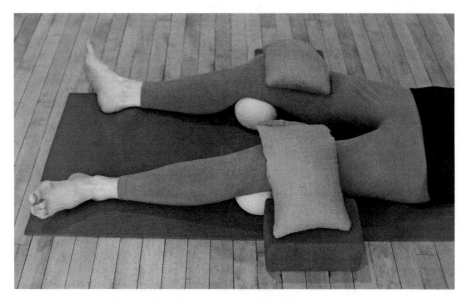

The Backs of the Knees with Added Weight

8. THE SACRUM

This one is a favorite for people who have a general achiness in the lower back. With a large, soft ball under the sacrum, you get a nice gentle stretch of your lumbar spine. It's calming after a long day of being on your feet, especially if you can rest your legs on a chair or couch.

Ball: One soft 5″–6″ ball

Body position: Lying on your back, legs bent. You can rest your feet on the floor, or lift them up as shown. You can also place your lower legs on a chair or couch.

Starting position of the ball: Under the middle of your sacrum

Action: Give yourself time to settle, and adjust the position of the ball as needed. Then begin to slowly explore small movements of your pelvis in any direction. The ball begins on the bony sacrum, but you can explore the edges of the bone and the surrounding muscles as well.

Progression: You can reach many good spots just by rolling, but you can also reposition the ball from time to time as desired.

Duration: 5–10 minutes

Contraindications: Sharp pain in the sacroiliac joint

Notes: If this technique is painful, start with the Back of the Pelvis technique from chapter 7.

Anatomy: Sacrum bone and associated ligaments

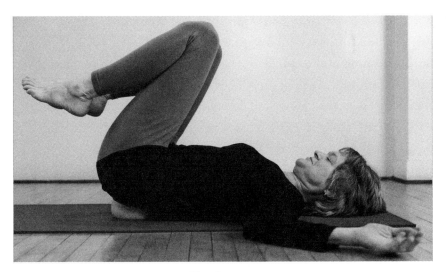

The Sacrum

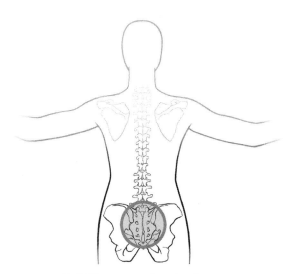

Ball Placement for the Sacrum

9. THE PELVIC FLOOR

The pelvic floor is a very sensitive area, and one that we don't usually explore other than for medical or sexual reasons. But pelvic floor disorders are surprisingly common, causing pain and urinary difficulties, and it is worth carefully exploring and revitalizing this area. There are several layers of muscles and fascia that can be tight or weak—or both tight *and* weak. Using the ball brings resilience to these tissues, and better functioning that can benefit your organ health, your elimination, your lower back, and your posture.

Ball: One soft 3″, 4″, or 5″ ball or the football-shaped ball

Body position: Sitting in a chair or on the floor

Starting position of the ball: Start with a spot that is not too sensitive.

Action: Sit still and breathe a few times to observe the sensations, then make very small pelvic movements in different directions. Use discretion and avoid extremely tender areas. Experiment with squeezing the ball with these muscles, and then releasing them.

Progression: Roll very slowly through the entire pelvic floor, from side to side, one sitting bone to the other, and also from front to back, from your pubic bone to your tailbone.

Duration: 3–5 minutes or more

Contraindications: Extreme sensitivity, recent childbirth or surgery

Notes: The fascia of the pelvic floor is continuous with the abdominal, hip, and lumbar fascia, forming a sling under the upper half of the body. You can combine this technique with ballwork on those areas to help release and invigorate the entire area.

Anatomy: Several layers of pelvic floor muscles, including piriformis, obturator internus, coccygeus, and levator ani

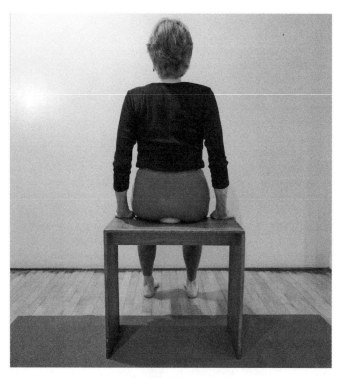

The Pelvic Floor

CHAPTER 14

The Lower Legs and Feet

As two-legged creatures, we depend on our feet for balance and locomotion. The foot has twenty-six bones and more than a dozen small muscles, but there are also muscles that span the distance between the knee and the sole of the foot that are involved with our every step. Those muscles are encased in fascial compartments, and that fascia can become overly tight, restricting circulation and movement range. The shoes we wear, the way we stand, the way we walk, and certainly the way we exercise—all affect the calves, ankles, and feet more than we might suspect. Inviting more awareness and circulation into your lower legs, ankles and feet can help develop better balance, better alignment of your ankles and feet, and a lighter and easier gait. If you have had an ankle sprain, collapsed arches, or plantar fasciitis, these techniques are very useful in the healing process. Remember to also practice the Soles of the Feet technique from chapter 7 as part of this lower leg and foot series.

1. THE CALVES

The two large muscles at the back of the calves work hard all day, propelling us forward in walking and running, and especially in jumping. Spasms or cramps in the legs can easily be remedied by regular work with the balls on these muscles. If you engage in sports frequently, drive for long periods of time, or stand at your job, your lower legs need this technique. If you have trouble winding down at the end of the day, this technique can help.
Balls: Two small 2.5″ solid balls

Body position: Lying on your back

Starting position of the balls: Just below the backs of your knees

Action: Spend a few minutes settling to allow your legs to relax over the balls. Find your "home base" position, which might be with your legs slightly turned out and might be different on each leg. Then begin to slowly turn your legs in toward the midline, back to home base, then out away from the midline, and back to home base again. Do this several times.

Progression: Move the balls a few inches down your calves. Repeat the same slow rotation of the legs, to cross-friction the muscles. Progress incrementally down your calves until you reach your Achilles tendon.

Duration: 10-15 minutes

Contraindications: Recent Achilles tendon tear

Notes: This is a wonderful one to do at the end of your day. Notice the feeling in your feet when you finish. For more pressure, cross one leg over the other.

Anatomy: Gastrocnemius, soleus, deep toe flexors, Achilles tendon, and all fascial layers

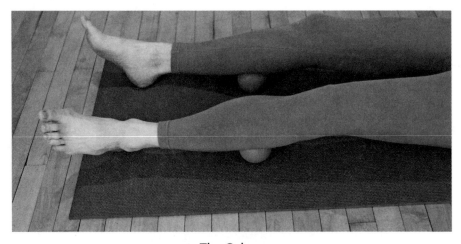

The Calves

2. THE FRONT SHINS

The muscle just to the outer side of the shinbone is the tibialis anterior. Its action is dorsiflexion, which occurs as you reach your heel forward and lift your toes to take a step. When this muscle becomes swollen after exertion (hiking, jumping on a hard surface, driving for long hours), the pain is sharp and deep because the swollen muscle is pressing nerves against the bone. This technique is intense and requires full knee flexion, but it can be done in short stints with intervals of time without the balls. A variation requiring less knee flexion is described below.

Balls: Two or four small 1"–2" hollow or solid balls

Body position: Kneeling on a mat with your feet folded under you or to the side of your hips, possibly with a block under your hips

Starting position of the balls: Near the top of your shinbones, just below the knees. For less intensity, sit on a block and use two balls on each leg to spread the contact area. For more intensity, use one ball on each leg and lean forward onto your arms.

Action: Move very slowly from side to side to cross-friction the muscles and fascia.

Progression: Working on one spot at a time, progress down your legs to just above your ankles. Take a break to stretch your ankles and knees whenever you need it.

Duration: 5–10 minutes

Contraindications: Recent knee or ankle injury

Variations: If the body position pictured here is difficult for you due to knee restrictions, experiment to find variations. For instance, you could stand beside a chair with a mat placed on the seat. Place the ball on the chair seat, and your tibialis anterior on the ball. Hold the chair with your hands, and move slowly over the ball, massaging the outer shin.

Anatomy: Tibialis anterior, extensor hallucis longus, extensor digitorum longus, peroneals, and all fascial layers

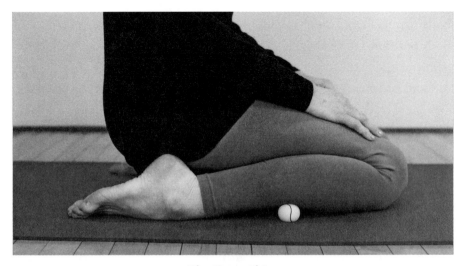

The Front Shins

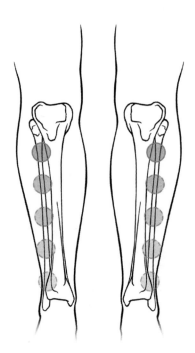

Ball Placement for the Front Shins

3. THE INNER AND OUTER CALVES

The sides of the calves can surprise you with trigger points and dull achi-ness. Working on this area improves the circulation and movement range in your ankles and feet. There are several variations, allowing you to control the intensity. The outer shin tends to be more dense and tight, but the inner calf can carry tension as well, and may be more sensitive.

Balls: Two balls, hollow or solid, 2″-4″, plus one 4″-5″ ball

Body position: Lie on your side with appropriate support for your spine. I rec-ommend a folded blanket or small pillow under your side ribs, and a higher support for your neck and head, leaving a space between the two supports for your shoulder. Your legs are in front of you with your knees bent and your legs separated to allow the balls access to the outer calf of the bottom leg and the inner calf of the top leg.

Starting position of the balls: There are several variations; see below.

Action: Move very slowly, exploring both a lengthwise movement of the ball along the muscles, and also a cross-friction action by slightly bending and straightening your knees.

Progression: Move the balls gradually down your calves to just above your ankles.

Duration: 10 minutes

Contraindications: None

Variations of ball placement:

1. Place one ball under the outer calf of the bottom leg, the other ball under the inner calf of the top leg, both near the knee. Try both the 2″ and 4″ size to determine your preference.

2. For more pressure on the outer shin of the bottom leg, stack your legs and possibly place a 4″ or 5″ ball between your knees. Place two small balls under your bottom calf. Continue to move in the same way, progressing down your leg. This position will simultaneously create more weight for the bottom leg and some good massage for the inner calf of both legs. Move the balls slowly down your legs in small increments.

3. Sit on the floor with one leg bent and one leg straight and to the side. Work with the ball under the outer shin of the bent leg, and lean into it with your hands for more pressure.

Anatomy: Inner gastrocnemius, peroneals, and all fascia layers

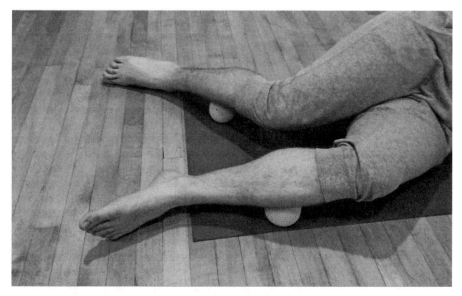

The Inner and Outer Calves 1

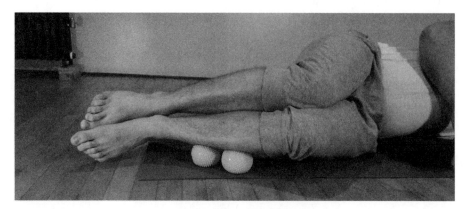

The Outer Calves 2

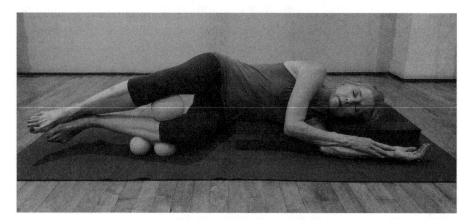

The Inner and Outer Calves 2

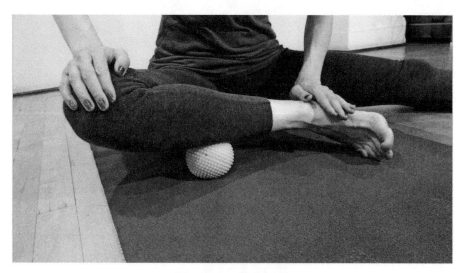

The Outer Calves 3

4. THE OUTER ANKLE AND FOOT

The outer edge of the ankle and foot is our fine-tuning balance support. Try standing on one leg for a few seconds, and watch this area responding to each small weight shift. Tightness here can force excess weight onto the inner edge of the foot, and over time, the arches will weaken. Working here can give us refined awareness and mobility that will greatly improve balance, and it can also heal a sprained ankle, once you can tolerate the pressure.

Johanna, the piano teacher you met earlier, was experiencing cramps in her lower legs and feet during the night when she moved her toes or her ankles. The cramps were worse on her right leg, the one she uses for the pedal under the piano. The cramps also coincided with the beginning of summer, when she started to wear sandals. There were many causative factors but one remedy: She tried this technique and found sensitive trigger points in her outer ankle and shin. After one concentrated session with this technique, the cramps ceased.

Ball: One 2″–4″ ball, either hollow or solid

Body position: Sitting on the floor with one leg bent, the other extended to the side. Put some support under your hips if needed.

Starting position of the ball: Under your outer ankle

Action: The movement is a combination of small movements initiated from your foot and ankle, combined with a guiding action with your hands. Also use your hands to give more pressure, and keep your tempo slow and steady. Explore all possible movements.

Progression: Move the ball incrementally along the outer edge of your foot, from around the ankle to the little toe. Work each spot patiently and slowly, adding pressure with your hands as you wish.

Repeat on the other side.

Duration: 5-10 minutes

Contraindications: Hip or knee restrictions that prevent sitting in this position

Notes: For more pressure, try this on the front foot in Pigeon Pose (one leg bent and forward and the other leg extending straight back behind you).

You can combine this technique with working on the top of the foot, as in the next technique. You may want to use a 3″–4″ ball on the outer ankle, and continue with a 1″–2″ ball on the foot.

Anatomy: Ankle retinaculum (band of connective tissue organizing the tendons of many muscles as they cross the ankle), tarsal and metatarsal bones, attachments of the peroneal muscles, and toe extensors

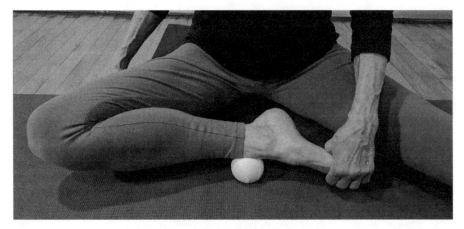

The Outer Ankle and Foot

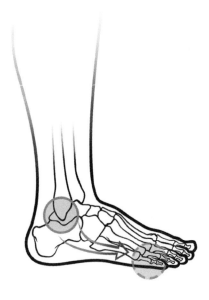

Ball Placement for the Outer Ankle and Foot

5. THE TOP OF THE FOOT (VERSION 1)

There are two ways to access the tops of your feet with the balls. Version 1 is sitting on the floor with support under your hips if needed, and your legs spread wide apart, as in the previous technique. You'll work on one foot at a time, and you'll need to get the top of your foot turned toward the floor and the sole of your foot facing upward, which involves rotating your leg. If that is not possible, you can try version 2 below, also for the top of the foot, but with a different sitting position.

You may not think there are any muscles on the tops of your feet—they feel very bony when you touch them—so why would we work there with the balls? In fact, you have muscles between the metatarsal bones that spread your toes, and also the toe extensor muscles, some of which are only in the foot, while others extend all the way up almost to your knees. When these muscles are tight, they can contribute to ankle stiffness, poor walking patterns, and even plantar fasciitis. The plantar fascia is spread across the bottoms of your feet and provides support for your arches and the muscles located there. Plantar fasciitis has many possible causes (poor arch support and weak feet are the most common), and one contributing factor can be chronic tension in the tops of the feet.

Judy, the health researcher you met earlier, has suffered from chronic plantar fasciitis and foot cramps for many years. After I taught her this technique, she had very direct and immediate relief. There was no need for surgery or drugs—just a few minutes on the balls.

Ball: One small 1"-2" ball, hollow or solid

Body position: Sitting on a blanket or two with one knee bent to the side, and the foot directly in front of you with the sole of the foot facing upward. The other leg can be in any comfortable position.

Starting position of the ball: Under the top of the foot of the bent leg

Action: Spend a few minutes adjusting to the seated position. If your bent leg does not rest easily on the floor, lean to that side until it does come down. You can turn the lower leg so that the sole of the foot faces upward.

Progression: Place the ball under your metatarsals—the part of your foot between your toes and your ankle. Press down into your foot with your hand to get the degree of pressure that you like. Then move your foot with your hand very slowly over the ball. You can move to different spots as desired, and do any manipulation of the foot (twisting, for example) that applies a good pressure into the metatarsal area.

Duration: 5 minutes per foot

Contraindications: Recent foot injury, hip or knee problems that prevent sitting on the floor

Anatomy: Toe extensor muscles, dorsal interossei muscles

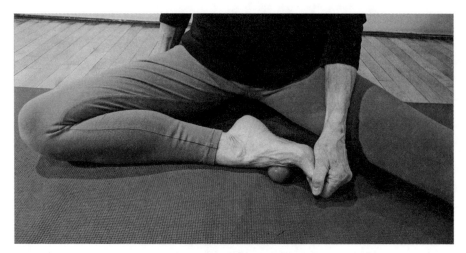

The Top of the Foot (Version 1)

6. THE TOPS OF THE FEET (VERSION 2)

Each step we take involves movement of the many joints in the foot. We instinctively coordinate the ankle, foot, and toes as we roll through the foot in a normal gait. Poor alignment, weak feet, or poor shoes (or all of the above) can derail this daily movement and cause pain and stiffness through the big toe and into the ankle. This technique brings relief and better ankle mobility, and more spring in your arches.

This technique is done in a kneeling position, with your feet and lower legs folded to the sides of your hips as in the yoga pose called Virasana. Sit on one or two blocks for support, and turn the soles of your feet upward, and the tops of your feet down toward the floor. If your knees are unhappy in this position, use version 1 above to work on the tops of the feet. In version 2, you can work with both feet at once, or one foot at a time by bringing the other leg forward in any comfortable position.

Balls: Two hollow 4" balls

Body position: Sitting on a block or other support, with one or both knees bent and feet pointing backward beside the hips, with the soles of the feet facing up.

Starting position of the balls: Under the tops of the feet

Action: Spend a few minutes adjusting to the seated position. If your knees are uncomfortable, sit on a higher support. Move your feet slowly over the balls, one at a time, or both feet at once. Use your hands to guide the movements of your feet and to give more pressure if desired.

Progression: Reposition the balls to reach every part of the foot and ankle.

Duration: 5 minutes per foot

Contraindications: Recent foot injury, hip or knee problems that prevent sitting in this position

Anatomy: Tibialis anterior, toe extensor muscles, dorsal interossei muscles, retinaculum, extensor hallucis longus, tarsal and metatarsal bones

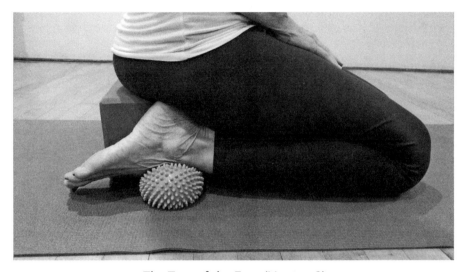

The Tops of the Feet (Version 2)

7. THE LEG NUTCRACKER

This one may make you laugh or cry! It's intense but worth trying, and works on the three hamstrings and the gastrocnemius/soleus muscles all at once. You can picture this action as separating strands of long muscles that have become stuck together. It's a "fast track" release for the backs of the legs.

Balls: Two 2″-4″ balls, hollow or solid

Body position: Sitting on your heels, toes pointed back, with padding under your legs as needed and possibly a block under your hips (the same position as in the previous technique). Lean forward onto your hands.

Starting position of the balls: Behind the knees, as far up as you can fit them

Action: At first, give yourself time to adjust to the pressure and choose whether to lean forward (gentler) or sit more upright (more intense). Then move your legs and hips very slowly from side to side, cross-frictioning the muscles.

Progression: One spot at a time, move the balls down your legs until you reach your ankles. In each spot, move your legs very slowly from side to side.

Duration: 5-10 minutes

Contraindications: Inability to sit in this position

Notes: Be sure to sit in the same position without the balls before you put the balls in, and after you take them out. The difference may surprise you!

Anatomy: Hamstrings, gastrocnemius, soleus, deep toe flexors

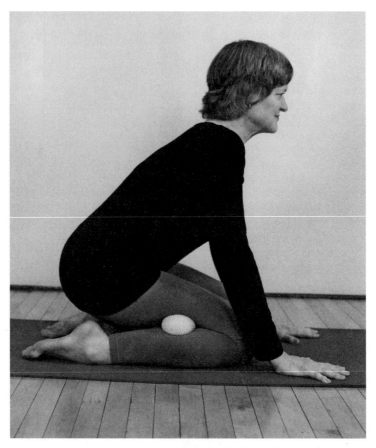

The Leg Nutcracker

CHAPTER 15

Conclusion

Embodied self-awareness is as fundamental to our survival and well-being as breathing and eating; it helps us self-monitor, self-regulate, and respond flexibly and adaptively in the present moment. To maintain our well-being throughout our lives, we must actively cultivate embodied self-awareness.[1]

People say that what we are all seeking is a meaning for life. I don't think that's what we're really seeking. I think that what we're really seeking is an experience of being alive, so that our life experience on the purely physical plane will have resonances within our innermost being and reality so that we actually feel the rapture of being alive.[2]

Holistic systems for bodymind reeducation and personal growth clearly have a place in the frameworks of both education and health care; in fact, they bridge the gap between other systems such as traditional and alternative medicine, psychotherapy, and fitness programs. Through a contemplative and therapeutic practice such as Bodymind Ballwork, you can gain new information and understanding in a direct and personal way about how to relieve pain, improve body mechanics, release held emotions, and increase mental clarity—and have a good time doing it. The in-depth discoveries that await us can connect to all aspects of our lives.

Because our modern culture as yet does not support an ongoing study of bodymind functioning, many of us may find ourselves overwhelmed by our own confusing array of tensions, pains, and stressors. We often don't know which aspects of ourselves most need to improve in order for our lives to improve. Do we need psychotherapy or physical therapy? Chiropractic or a dance class? Elsa Gindler and those who followed her saw that this quandary could be solved only by a holistic approach that acknowledges the interconnectedness of our emotional, intellectual, sensory, and movement selves.

An apt analogy for this idea of a holistic approach appears in Edward Maisel's introduction to his collection of the writings of F. M. Alexander, the founder of the Alexander Technique. He compares working with the entire bodymind—instead of one symptom at a time—to cleaning up a messy room in order to find a lost object, rather than looking for the object amid the mess:

> The indirect way . . . may take a little longer, but it is more certain, will render further losses less likely, and will have accomplished something useful even if the missing object remains unfound. Also it may happen that something lost long since and which has been forgotten may turn up. It has, too, the further important advantage that one will at last become fully aware of the contents of the room in a way that one had not been before.[3]

This holistic view of human consciousness brings us back to the koshas—the five layers of being from the yoga tradition. Let's review the five koshas from chapter 1. The first, the outermost layer, is made up of the physical tissues of the body, the "body of food"; the second one is the "body of breath"; the third one is the mental processes, the "body of thoughts"; the fourth one, the "wisdom body"; and the fifth one, the "body of bliss" (see illustration on page fourteen). This conceptual map identifies human consciousness in different forms. Each layer is more subtle than the one before, yet they are all available to us. As we go through our life journey, we touch on each of these parts of ourselves repeatedly, both in the smallest moments of daily life and in the times of deepest meaning.

In body therapies, we start with the outermost layer because it is the easiest one to access. We all can feel hot and cold, pain and pleasure, hunger and thirst, and the basic movements of daily life. For some, that's as far as body awareness goes. We're lucky if we even feel ourselves breathing. Then there are athletes, dancers, actors, and musicians, who develop a more refined awareness of the interaction between body and mind necessary to refine their skills and their performance. But to go even deeper than that, and to discover what's inside the "room" of our inner being, we need a slow, contemplative technique like Bodymind Ballwork. Through this kind of intentional internal focus, we can develop an authentic connection with our posture and our movement habits, our breath, and how our thoughts and emotions become part of the body's physical structure. Knowledge arises spontaneously when we are in touch with the body. I like to think of Bodymind Ballwork as a "body meditation." Just as we might use a mantra or the rhythm of the breath to carry our awareness inside, the balls serve that purpose in this method. Insights arise when we contact a deep part of ourselves. With embodied self-awareness, we have a gateway into more self-understanding, a built-in protection from physical strains, and a greater flexibility in responding to everyday challenges.

Embodied self-awareness might not be attained through a linear learning process; changes and improvements may come slowly sometimes, or with surprising speed at other times. When you least expect it, your bodymind might be ready for positive change. Whereas some bodymind techniques require that students discontinue their poor movement habits before better patterns are attempted in a set sequence, Bodymind Ballwork allows for a high degree of individual autonomy and a fluid process in moving from old habits to new ones. There is no set sequence of techniques; each practitioner discovers what works best for him or her. The new sensations made possible by the balls give the practitioner a chance to renew and refresh body awareness moment by moment, and to replace old patterns with new and more healthy patterns little by little, one practice at a time. We work from an investigative frame of mind, staying in the present moment to feel the body and respond to the pressure of the ball.

What we learn, from connecting with ongoing sensations inside the body and simple movement, is kinesthetic literacy, a knowledge of our particular movement style and capacity. As our kinesthetic sense becomes more refined, we move more intelligently, and we also see that physical sensations begin to evoke new patterns of thought. Whereas we may have reacted to the pain of a strained muscle with feelings of frustration and fear, we now can listen to what the body is asking for. We can quiet the mind's usual chatter, and stay with sensations that are happening right now, rather than the memory or fear of pain from the past. And when the ballwork feels good, that pleasure is entrancing and restorative at a very deep level.

One student said, "It's about doing away with the self-destructive devil that lives within all of us. . . . The more you do it, the more aware you become, like peeling away layer after layer of debris, and really finding more and more understanding, awareness, and inner knowledge. Not assumed knowledge, but the innate knowledge."

I envision this kind of exploration and self-study becoming an integral part of education at every level, with playful opportunities for children to develop kinesthetic literacy and pleasure from embodied self-awareness. Research shows that children learn best with an element of active physical participation—less sitting at desks, more moving through the learning process. This work gives familiar rubber balls a whole new realm of meaning as an interactive tool for growth.

Bodymind techniques are already vital components of dance and drama training, helping performers to develop their expressive range through embodied self-awareness. Actors develop refinements that allow their whole bodies to express their role more fully. Dancers need this kind of work to avert injuries or recover from them, and to counteract the repetitive movements inherent in hours and hours of rehearsal. But beyond the healing aspect of the work, Bodymind Ballwork will enable a higher level of authentic physical expression for any performer. Mark, a dancer who works daily with the balls, says that in his embodied state, his body is totally integrated, and dancing is effortless, fluid, and ecstatic.

In psychotherapy, and particularly trauma recovery, balls can provide a safe companion in the work of processing emotional experiences that are held in the tissues. You can explore at your own pace, in private or with a teacher, and gradually build a meaningful connection to your body as a source of deep knowledge and support.

In my experience, this work is most meaningful to those who can suspend their judgments of their body enough to experiment and play, to trust that the body has wisdom to impart. Kinesthetic literacy doesn't come from studying anatomy (although that study can be empowering as well); it is learned by doing, by moving. As Gindler said, "To know is not enough. You must do it."[4]

As you practice, I encourage you to remember the basic principles:

1. **Develop awareness without judgment.** Give yourself the gift of attention to your inner sensations without rushing to judgment, solutions, or analysis.

2. **Release into gravity.** Let the floor and the balls fully support you. Letting go is a skill worth practicing. Allow the pressure of the balls to elicit relaxation as you drape yourself over them.

3. **Move slowly with minimal effort.** You will feel more subtlety if you move slowly, and your soft tissues will have the time they need to respond to the ball's pressure.

4. **Explore your range.** Try different directions of movement, knowing that support from the ball could open up new possibilities, new freedom.

The process is simple, the tools are simple, but the rewards are profound. Becoming more in touch with yourself physically and emotionally is the most worthwhile self-care there is. You will feel better, move better, think more clearly, and be more available and resilient in your work and your relationships. You may find that you naturally make better choices that support your own health, because your mind and the body are authentically connected. The process of healing and inner growth is ongoing, and it is a fascinating, ever-new adventure. I invite you to use this book as your guide, develop your inner resources, and build your own well-being from the inside out.

NOTES

INTRODUCTION

1 Elsa Gindler, "Gymnastik for Busy People," *Sensory Awareness Bulletin: Elsa Gindler 1885–1961* 1, no. 10 (Summer 1978): 40.

2 Mirka Knaster, *Discovering the Body's Wisdom* (New York: Bantam Books, 1996), 352–380.

3 Alan Fogel, *Body Sense: The Science and Practice of Embodied Self-Awareness* (New York: W. W. Norton, 2013), 29–33.

4 Fogel, *Body Sense,* xi.

5 Bessel van der Kolk, *The Body Keeps the Score* (New York: Penguin Books, 2014), 275.

6 Gindler, "Gymnastik for Busy People," 36–40.

CHAPTER 1: THE BODYMIND CONNECTION

1 Robert M. Sapolsky, *Why Zebras Don't Get Ulcers* (New York: St. Martin's Griffin, 1994).

2 John Grimes, *A Concise Dictionary of Indian Philosophy* (Albany: State University of New York Press, 1996), 167.

3 Ivy Green, *Relaxation Awareness Resilience: Rosen Method Bodywork Science and Practice* (Campbell, CA: Fast Pencil, 2016), 230–231.

CHAPTER 2: THE NERVOUS SYSTEM, STRESS, AND RELAXATION

1 "Recent work by the psychologist Shelley Taylor of UCLA has forced people to rethink this. She suggests that the fight-or-flight response is what dealing with stress is about in males, and that it has been overemphasized as a phenomenon

because of the long-standing bias among (mostly male) scientists to study males rather than females.

Taylor argues convincingly that the physiology of the stress-response can be quite different in females, built around the fact that in most species, females are typically less aggressive than males, and that having dependent young often precludes the option of flight. Showing that she can match the good old boys at coming up with a snappy sound-bite, Taylor suggests that rather than the female stress-response being about fight-or-flight, it's about "tend and befriend"—taking care of her young and seeking social affiliation." (Sapolsky, *Why Zebras Don't Get Ulcers*, 33)

2   Grimes, *A Concise Dictionary of Indian Philosophy*, 167.

3   Green, *Relaxation Awareness Resilience*, 196.

4   The hypothalamus starts the process of activation of the stress response, which is both neurological and hormonal. Our central stress response system is called the HPA axis, and it goes like this: the hypothalamus sends the hormone corticotropin releasing factor (CRF) to the pituitary gland, which secretes adrenocorticotropic hormone (ACTH), which tells the adrenal glands to secrete cortisol and epinephrine. This axis was first described by Hans Selye.

5   Homeostasis is the process of maintaining balance in the body's physiological functions.

6   Sapolsky, *Why Zebras Don't Get Ulcers*, 48–49.

7   Green, *Relaxation Awareness Resilience*, 125–128.

8   Herbert Benson, *The Relaxation Response* (New York: HarperCollins, 1975).

9   Green, *Relaxation Awareness Resilience*, 196.

10   Mel Robin, *A Handbook for Yogasana Teachers: The Incorporation of Neuroscience, Physiology, and Anatomy into the Practice* (Tucson, AZ: Wheatmark, 2009), 179–182.

CHAPTER 3: SOFT TISSUES, PAIN, AND RELEASE

1   "The definition of the word 'fascia' is evolving; researchers and clinicians don't always agree on what types of tissue are included in this term. Some include ligaments, tendons, aponeuroses, joint capsules, and retinacula as 'fascia,' seeing it from a broader functional point of view." (David Lesondak, *Fascia: What It Is and Why It Matters*, Edinburgh: Handspring, 2017, 1)

2   Thomas W. Findley and Robert Schleip, eds., *Fascia Research: Basic Science and Implications for Conventional and Complementary Health Care* (Munich: Elsevier, 2007).

3   Ibid., 157–158.

4   Thomas W. Myers, *Anatomy Trains: Myofascial Meridians for Manual and Movement Therapists* (Edinburgh: Elsevier, 2014), 301.

5   Lesondak, *Fascia*, 11.

6 Fogel, *Body Sense*, 193.

7 Robert Schleip, "Fascia as a Sensory Organ," in *Dynamic Body: Myoskeletal Alignment: Exploring Form, Expanding Function*, ed. Erik Dalton (Oklahoma City, OK: Freedom from Pain Institute, 2012), 137-163.

CHAPTER 4: BODY SCHEMA, BODY IMAGE, AND CONDITIONING

1 Paul Schilder, *The Image and Appearance of the Human Body* (New York: International Universities Press, 1978), 112.

2 This condition, which also can occur in those with normal childhoods, has various medical names: tactile defensiveness, sensory processing disorder, sensory integration dysfunction.

3 Fogel, *Body Sense*, 195.

4 Green, *Relaxation Awareness Resilience*, 128; Rick Hanson with Richard Mendius, *Buddha's Brain* (Oakland, CA: New Harbinger, 2009), 67-77.

5 Green, *Relaxation Awareness Resilience*, 299.

6 Daniel J. Siegel and Tina Payne Bryson, *The Whole-Brain Child* (New York: Bantam Books, 2011), 72.

7 Donna Jackson Nakazawa, *Childhood Disrupted: How Your Biography Becomes Your Biology and How You Can Heal* (New York: Atria/Simon & Schuster, 2016).

8 Epigenetics is the study of how a gene's expression and function can be dynamically altered by environmental factors.

CHAPTER 5: DEFENSE MECHANISMS AND TRAUMA

1 Green, *Relaxation Awareness Resilience*, 75.

2 Paolo Tozzi, "Does Fascia Hold Memories?" *Journal of Bodywork and Movement Therapies* 18, no. 2: 259-265.

3 Bessel van der Kolk, quoted in Green, *Relaxation Awareness Resilience*, 327.

4 van der Kolk, *The Body Keeps the Score*, 4.

5 Fogel, *Body Sense*, 58.

6 Siegel and Bryson, *The Whole-Brain Child*, 37-61.

7 Note: other writers refer to these two ways of functioning as "bottom up" and "top down." See Hanson, *Buddha's Brain*, 107-108.

8 Fogel, *Body Sense*, 56.

9 Hanson, *Buddha's Brain*, 101.

10 These areas are the anterior cingulate cortex motor area and the supplementary motor area.

11 James Austin, quoted in Green, *Relaxation Awareness Resilience*, 367.

12 Fogel, *Body Sense*, 95-101.

13 van der Kolk, quoted in Green, *Relaxation Awareness Resilience*, 284.

14 Ibid., 337-338.

15 van der Kolk, *The Body Keeps the Score*, 333.

16 Ibid., 357.

17 Green, *Relaxation Awareness Resilience*, 278-279.

CHAPTER 15: CONCLUSION

1 Green, *Relaxation Awareness Resilience*, 270.

2 Joseph Campbell, quoted in Green, *Relaxation Awareness Resilience*, 355.

3 Edward Maisel, introduction to *The Resurrection of the Body: The Essential Writings of F. Matthias Alexander*, ed. Edward Maisel (Boston: Shambhala, 1969), xxx.

4 Gindler, "Gymnastik for Busy People," 4.

BIBLIOGRAPHY

BOOKS

Alexander, F. Matthias. *The Resurrection of the Body: The Essential Writings of F. Matthias Alexander.* Selected and introduced by Edward Maisel. Boston: Shambhala, 1969.

Benson, Herbert. *The Relaxation Response.* New York: HarperCollins, 1975.

Bertherat, Therese, and Carol Bernstein. *The Body Has Its Reasons.* New York: Random House, Pantheon Books, 1977.

Biel, Andrew. *Trail Guide to the Body.* Boulder, CO: Books of Discovery, 2014.

—— *Trail Guide to Movement: Building the Body in Motion.* Boulder, CO: Books of Discovery, 2015.

Blakeslee, Sandra, and Matthew Blakeslee. *The Body Has a Mind of Its Own.* New York: Random House, 2008.

Brooks, Charles V. W. *Sensory Awareness: The Rediscovery of Experiencing.* New York: Viking Press, 1974.

Cobb, Elissa. *The Forgotten Body.* Hardwick, MA: Satya House, 2008.

Dalton, Erik, ed. *Dynamic Body: Myoskeletal Alignment: Exploring Form, Expanding Function.* Oklahoma City, OK: Freedom from Pain Institute, 2012.

Damasio, Antonio. *The Feeling of What Happens.* New York: Houghton Mifflin Harcourt, 1999.

—— *Self Comes to Mind.* New York: Random House, 2010.

Doidge, Norman. *The Brain That Changes Itself.* New York: Penguin Books, 2007.

—— *The Brain's Way of Healing.* New York: Penguin Books, 2015.

Dychtwald, Ken. *Bodymind.* New York: Harcourt Brace Jovanovich/Jove Publications, 1977.

Earls, James, and Thomas Myers. *Fascial Release for Structural Balance.* Berkeley, CA: North Atlantic Books, 2010.

Feldenkrais, Moshe. *Awareness through Movement.* New York: Harper and Row, 1972.

—— *Body and Mature Behavior: A Study of Anxiety, Sex, Gravitation, and Learning.* New York: International Universities Press, 1979.

Findley, Thomas W., and Robert Schleip, eds. *Fascia Research: Basic Science and Implications for Conventional and Complementary Health Care.* Munich: Elsevier, 2007.

Fogel, Alan. *Body Sense: The Science and Practice of Embodied Self-Awareness.* New York: W. W. Norton, 2013.

Green, Ivy. *Relaxation Awareness Resilience: Rosen Method Bodywork Science and Practice.* Campbell, CA: Fast Pencil, 2016.

Grimes, John. *A Concise Dictionary of Indian Philosophy.* Albany: State University of New York Press, 1996.

Hanson, Rick, with Richard Mendius. *Buddha's Brain.* Oakland, CA: New Harbinger, 2009.

Johnson, Don Hanlon, ed. *Bone, Breath & Gesture: Practices of Embodiment.* Berkeley, CA: North Atlantic Books, 1995.

Johnson, Don Hanlon. *The Protean Body.* New York: Harper and Row, 1977.

Knaster, Mirka. *Discovering the Body's Wisdom.* New York: Bantam Books, 1996.

Lesondak, David. *Fascia: What It Is and Why It Matters.* Edinburgh: Handspring, 2017.

Lindsay, Mark. *Fascia: Clinical Applications for Health and Human Performance.* Clifton Park, NY: Delmar Cengage Learning, 2008.

Myers, Thomas W. *Anatomy Trains: Myofascial Meridians for Manual and Movement Therapists.* Edinburgh: Elsevier, 2014.

——. *The Anatomist's Corner: Collected Articles: Issues in Structural Anatomy.* Walpole, ME: Kinesis, 2014.

—— *Body³: A Therapist's Anatomy Reader.* Walpole, ME: Kinesis, 2014.

Nakazawa, Donna Jackson. *Childhood Disrupted: How Your Biography Becomes Your Biology and How You Can Heal.* New York: Atria/Simon & Schuster, 2016.

Pert, Candace B. *Molecules of Emotion.* New York: Scribner, 2003.

Robin, Mel. *A Handbook for Yogasana Teachers: The Incorporation of Neuroscience, Physiology, and Anatomy into the Practice.* Tucson, AZ: Wheatmark, 2009.

Saltonstall, Ellen. *Anatomy and Yoga: A Guide for Teachers and Students.* New York: Abhyasa Press, 2016.

Sapolsky, Robert M. *Why Zebras Don't Get Ulcers.* New York: St. Martin's Griffin, 1994.

Schilder, Paul. *The Image and Appearance of the Human Body.* New York: International Universities Press, 1978.

Schleip, Robert, ed. *Fascia in Sport and Movement.* East Lothian, Scotland: Handspring, 2015.

Schleip, Robert. *Fascial Fitness.* Chichester, UK: Lotus, 2017.

Schleip, Robert, Thomas W. Findley, Leon Chaitow, and Peter A. Huijing, eds. *Fascia: The Tensional Network of the Human Body.* Edinburgh: Elsevier, 2012.

Schultz, R. Louis, and Rosemary Feitis. *The Endless Web: Fascial Anatomy and Physical Reality.* Berkeley, CA: North Atlantic Books, 1996.

Siegel, Daniel J., and Tina Payne Bryson. *The Whole-Brain Child.* New York: Bantam Books, 2011.

Speads, Carola H. *Ways to Better Breathing.* Great Neck, NY: Felix Morrow, 1986.

Todd, Mabel Elsworth. *The Thinking Body.* New York: Dance Horizons, 1968.

van Der Kolk, Bessel. *The Body Keeps the Score: Brain, Mind, and Body in the Healing of Trauma.* New York: Penguin Books, 2013.

JOURNAL ARTICLES

Comeaux, Z. "Dynamic Fascial Release and the Role of Mechanical/Vibrational Assist Devices in Manual Therapies." [Review]. *Journal of Bodywork and Movement Therapies* 15, no. 1 (2011): 35–41. https://doi:10.1016/j.jbmt.2010.02.006.

Danner, Ursula, et al. "ABC–The Awareness-Body-Chart: A New Tool Assessing Body Awareness." *PLOS One*, 2017. https://doi.org/10.1371/journal.pone.0186597.

Gulick, D. T., K. Palombaro, et al. "Effect of Ischemic Pressure Using a Backnobber II Device on Discomfort Associated with Myofascial Trigger Points." *Journal of Bodywork and Movement Therapies* 15, no. 3 (2011): 319–325.

LeBauer, A., R. Brtalik, and K. Stowe. "The Effect of Myofascial Release (MFR) on an Adult with Idiopathic Scoliosis." [Case Reports]. *Journal of Bodywork and Movement Therapies* 12, no. 4 (2008): 356–363. https://doi:10.1016/j.jbmt.2008.03.008.

Mehling, Wolf E., Viranjini Gopisetty, Jennifer Daubenmier, Cynthia J. Price, Frederick M. Heckt, and Anita Steward. "Body Awareness: Construct and Self-Report Measures." *PLOS One*, 2009. https://doi.org/10.1371/journal.pone.0005614.

Sensory Awareness Foundation (formerly Charlotte Selver Foundation). *Sensory Awareness: The Work of Selver.* Caldwell, NJ: 1973.

——, *Sensory Awareness Bulletin: Elsa Gindler 1885–1961* 1, no. 10 (Summer 1978).

——, *Sensory Awareness Bulletin: Elsa Gindler 1885–1961* II, no. 10 (Winter 1981).

——, *Sensory Awareness Bulletin: Elsa Gindler 1885–1961* no. 11 (Winter 1983).

Tozzi, Paolo. "Does Fascia Hold Memories?" *Journal of Bodywork and Movement Therapies* 18, no. 2 (2014): 259–265.

Tozzi, P., D. Bongiorno, and C. Vitturini. "Fascial Release Effects on Patients with Non-specific Cervical or Lumbar Pain." [Clinical Trial]. *Journal of Bodywork and Movement Therapies* 15, no. 4 (2011): 405–416. https://doi:10.1016/j.jbmt.2010.11.003.

Whitaker, Robert C., et al. "Adverse Childhood Experiences, Dispositional Mindfulness, and Adult Health." *Preventive Medicine*, 2014. https://doi:10.1016/j.ypmed.2014.07.029.

ABOUT THE AUTHOR

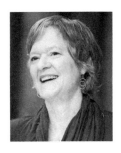 ELLEN SALTONSTALL has been teaching yoga, anatomy, yoga therapeutics, and Bodymind Ballwork to improve wellness for people of all ages since 1985. Her background includes modern dance and massage therapy, both of which brought her to working with the balls for self-massage. Her previous titles include *Yoga for Arthritis* and *Yoga for Osteoporosis* (with Dr. Loren Fishman) and *Anatomy and Yoga: A Guide for Teachers and Students.* Saltonstall's writings have appeared in *Yoga Journal, Topics in Geriatric Rehabilitation,* and the International Association of Yoga Therapists' *International Journal of Yoga Therapy.*

Her yoga education stems from the Iyengar and Anusara traditions, with many master teachers over thirty-five years. She offers webinars with YogaUOnline on topics such as osteoporosis, joint health, back pain, and myofascial release. Currently she lives in New York City and teaches yoga, anatomy, yoga therapeutics, and Bodymind Ballwork to students and teachers internationally, inviting them to discover and explore the majesty and mystery of the human form.

For upcoming programs, courses, and webinars, please visit Saltonstall's website www.ellensaltonstall.com. To purchase balls, visit www.lifesaball.org and look for the Bodymind Ballwork page.

About North Atlantic Books

North Atlantic Books (NAB) is an independent, nonprofit publisher committed to a bold exploration of the relationships between mind, body, spirit, and nature. Founded in 1974, NAB aims to nurture a holistic view of the arts, sciences, humanities, and healing. To make a donation or to learn more about our books, authors, events, and newsletter, please visit www.northatlanticbooks.com.

North Atlantic Books is the publishing arm of the Society for the Study of Native Arts and Sciences, a 501(c)(3) nonprofit educational organization that promotes cross-cultural perspectives linking scientific, social, and artistic fields. To learn how you can support us, please visit our website.